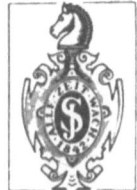

Recent Developments
in Lipid and Lipoprotein Research

H. U. Klör (Ed.)

Lipoprotein Subfractions Omega-3 Fatty Acids

With 48 Figures and 8 Tables

Springer-Verlag Berlin Heidelberg GmbH

Prof. Dr. med. H. U. Klör
Med. Zentrum für Innere Medizin
Med. Klinik III und Poliklinik
Universität Gießen
Rodthohl 6
6300 Gießen

ISBN 978-3-540-19146-9   ISBN 978-3-642-83447-9 (eBook)
DOI 10.1007/978-3-642-83447-9

Preface

On November 6 and 7, 1987, lipid and lipoprotein researchers from all over Europe convened in Munich on the occasion of the second European Workshop on Lipid Metabolism (EWLM). This informal gathering was devoted to two main topics, and recent research results were presented and discussed during a poster session.

Recent developments in the physiology and pathophysiology of lipoprotein subfractions were discussed on the first day of the meeting. In recent years, new analytical tools have been created for analyzing lipoprotein subfractions, particularly the apolipoprotein component. With the introduction of immunological and electrophoretic methods it has become clear that the heterogeneity of the plasma lipoprotein system is even greater than had been assumed only a decade or so ago. Despite this, it is apparent from the contributions to this volume that new methods for differentiating lipoprotein subfractions will increase our understanding of lipoprotein metabolism, especially of the triglyceride-rich lipoprotein particles and the high-density lipoproteins. The complex functions of the various plasma apolipoproteins and their association with the lipoprotein lipid in single or complex lipoprotein particles give rise to a complex and dynamic metabolic system that changes constantly during the day. While it has for some time been possible to delineate fairly accurately the atherogenic potential of low-density lipoproteins, which are comparatively simple lipoprotein particles, the new methods of lipoprotein subfraction analysis will be needed to select and differentiate amongst the potentially atherogenic triglyceride-rich particles, especially the chylomicron and very low density lipoprotein remnants. This lipoprotein subfraction analysis, combined with improved methods of analyzing the high-density lipoproteins, will allow atherogenic and non-atherogenic lipoprotein constellations to be discriminated and a more accurate prediction of an individual's risk of developing atherosclerotic vascular disease.

On the second day of the symposium, a relatively new aspect of lipid and lipoprotein metabolism was covered, namely the therapeutic role of ω_3-fatty acids derived from marine oils. This area of research has developed only recently, but it is rapidly expanding because of the widespread interest in this new form of therapy. We learned during the meeting that ω_3-fatty acids do not only influence lipid and lipoprotein metabolism but may, through their effect on platelet activity, also have an effect on thromboembolic complications of vascular disease. It also became clear that ω_3-fatty acids have a profound effect on cellular functions by altering membrane fluidity and, particularly, by modulating cellular prostanoid metabolism. It is in this latter field of research that the most progress will have to be expected in the years to come. Vast perspectives on new therapeutic applications are opening up in the area of immunological disorders such as autoimmune disease of various organ systems such as the skin, soft tissues inflammatory bowel disease etc. It is possible that ω_3-fatty acids will be used in the future as a basic and relatively innocuous means of immunomodulation in conjunction with classical immunomodulating agents as steroids and other anti-inflammatory drugs. As the contributions to this symposium clearly showed, the role of ω_3-fatty acids as a protective agent against the development of atherosclerotic vascular disease is not yet clear and further studies will have to provide more evidence in that direction.

Last but not least, the truly generous support of Fournier-Holphar, which made this very successful meeting possible, should be mentioned.

Gießen, FRG   Prof. Dr. H. U. Klör

Contents

Omega-3 Fatty Acids
Chairmen: R. Paoletti, G. Schlierf, and H. Canzler

List of Contributors

AILHAND, G.
  Centre de Biochimie, Faculté des Sciences, Parc Valrose, 06034 Nice Cedex, France

ALAUPOVIC, P.
  Oklahoma Medical Research Foundation, Oklahoma City, OK 73104, USA

AVOGARO, P.
  Ospedali Civili Venezia, Divisione Medica III, Centro Scientifico Regionale, Unità Operativa di Venezia, 30100 Venezia, Italy

BARD, J.M.
  Institut Pasteur, SERLIA, 1, rue du Professeur Calmette, 59019 Lille Cedex, France

BATES, D.
  Department of Neurology, University of Newcastle upon Tyne, Queen Victoria Road, Newcastle upon Tyne NE 1 4LP, U.K.

BERGSETH, S.
  Institute of Medical Biochemistry, University of Oslo, P.O. Box 1112, Blindern, 0317 Oslo 3, Norway

BREMER, J.
  Institute of Medical Biochemistry, University of Oslo, P.O. Box 1112, Blindern, 0317 Oslo 3, Norway

CROSET, M.
  CNRS UA 273, Université de Bourgogne, B.P. 138, 21004 Dijon, France

FRENCH, J.M.
  Department of Neurology, University of Newcastle upon Tyne, Queen Victoria Road, Newcastle upon Tyne NE1 4LP, U.K.

FRUCHART, J.C.

Institut Pasteur, SERLIA, 1, rue du Professeur Calmette, 59019 Lille Cedex, France

GALLI, C.

Institute of Pharmacological Sciences, University of Milan, 20100 Milan, Italy

HAWKINS, S.A.

Department of Medicine, Queen's University of Belfast, Belfast, U.K.

KAFFARNIK, H.

Abteilung für Endokrinologie und Stoffwechsel, Zentrum Innere Medizin der Philipps-Universität Marburg, Baldinger Straße, 3550 Marburg, W.-Germany

KLÖR, H.U.

Medizinisches Zentrum für Innere Medizin, Medizinische Klinik III und Poliklinik, Klinikum der Justus-Liebig-Universität Gießen, Rodthohl 6, 6300 Gießen, W.-Germany

KOSTNER, G.

Institut für Medizinische Biochemie, Universität Graz, Harrachgasse 21, 8010 Graz, Austria

LAGARDE, M.

Institut National des Sciences Appliquées de Lyon, 20, avenue Albert Einstein, 69621 Villeurbanne Cedex, France

LINN, TH.

Medizinisches Zentrum für Innere Medizin, Medizinische Klinik III und Poliklinik, Klinikum der Justus-Liebig-Universität Gießen, Rodthohl 6, 6300 Gießen, W.-Germany

LONTIE, J.-F.

Fondation de Recherche sur l'Athérosclérose Bruxelles, Université Libre de Bruxelles, 1000 Bruxelles, Belgium

LULEY, C.H.

Abteilung für Klinische Chemie und Laboratoriumsmedizin, Klinikum der Johannes-Gutenberg-Universität Mainz, Naunynweg, 6500 Mainz, W.-Germany

MADERNA, P.

Institute of Pharmacological Sciences, University of Milan, 20100 Milan, Italy

MALMENDIER, C.L.

Fondation de Recherche sur l'Athérosclérose Bruxelles, Université Libre de Bruxelles, 1000 Bruxelles, Belgium

PAOLETTI, R.
Institute of Pharmacological Sciences, University of Milan, 20100 Milan, Italy

ROBENEK, H.
Institut für Arterioskleroseforschung an der Universität Münster,
Domagkstraße 3, 4400 Münster, W.-Germany

SCHMITZ, G.
Institut für Klinische Chemie und Laboratoriumsmedizin, Universität Münster,
Albert-Schweitzer-Straße 33, 4400 Münster, W.-Germany

SHAW, D.A.
Department of Neurology, University of Newcastle upon Tyne,
Queen Victoria Road, Newcastle upon Tyne NE1 4 LP, U.K.

SIRTORI, C.R.
Center E. Grossi Paoletti, University of Milan, 20129 Milan, Italy

SMITH, A.D.
The Middlesex Hospital, London, U.K.

SMITH, S.
Department of Neurology, University of Newcastle upon Tyne,
Queen Victoria Road, Newcastle upon Tyne NE1 4LP, U.K.

SPYDEVOLD, Ø.
Institute of Medical Biochemistry, University of Oslo, P.O. Box 1112, Blindern,
0317 Oslo 3, Norway

STEINMETZ, A.
Institut Pasteur, SERLIA, 1, rue du Professeur Calmette, 59019 Lille Cedex,
France and Abteilung für Endokrinologie und Stoffwechsel,
Zentrum Innere Medizin der Philipps-Universität Marburg, Baldinger Straße,
3550 Marburg, W.-Germany

STEYRER, E.
Institut für Medizinische Biochemie, Universität Graz, Harrachgasse 21,
8010 Graz, Austria

THOMPSON, G.R.
Hammersmith Hospital, MRC Lipoprotein Team, London, U.K.

THOMPSON, R.H.S.
The Middlesex Hospital, London, U.K.

v. Tol, A.

Department of Biochemistry I, Erasmus University Rotterdam, P.O. Box 1738, 3000 DR Rotterdam, The Netherlands

Tremoli, E.

Institute of Pharmacological Sciences, University of Milan, 20100 Milan, Italy

Véricel, C.

CNRS UA 273, Université de Bourgogne, B.P. 138, 21004 Dijon, France

Wieland, H.

Medizinische Universitätsklinik der Universität Freiburg, Hugstetter Straße 55, 7800 Freiburg, W.-Germany

Wolfram, G.

Medizinische Poliklinik der Universität München, Pettenkoferstraße 8a, 8000 München 2

Woo, E.

Department of Neurology, University of Newcastle upon Tyne, Queen Victoria Road, Newcastle upon Tyne NE1 4LP, U.K.

Lipoprotein Subfractions;
Their Role in Lipid Transport and Atherosclerosis

Chairmen: W. F. RIESEN, G. C. DESCOVICH, H. KAFFARNIK,
P. DOUSTE-BLAZY, P. RUBBA, G. MANZATO, and A. VAN TOL

The Lipoprotein Family Concept: An Update

P. ALAUPOVIC

Since the early 1940s the classification of plasma lipoproteins has been based on their nonspecific physical properties such as hydrated density, size, and electric charge, and the operationally-defined lipoproteins have been considered to represent the fundamental chemical and metabolic entities of the lipid transport system [1]. However, more recently accumulated evidence has pointed out that this conceptual approach is untenable, because lipoprotein classes, defined by their physical properties, are both chemically and metabolically heterogeneous [2, 3]. In addition to hydrated density, size, and charge distribution, major operationally-defined lipoprotein classes are also heterogeneous with respect to their lipid/protein and apolipoprotein composition. The occurrence of apolipoproteins in non-equimolar ratios and the immunochemical patterns of non-identity or partial identity between at least some apolipoproteins have provided the crucial evidence that individual lipoprotein particles of the same density class cannot have the same apolipoprotein composition. Moreover, these findings have suggested that the operationally-defined lipoprotein classes consist of several distinct lipoprotein species rather than a single homogeneous lipid/protein complex [2, 4, 5]. The recently established kinetic heterogeneity of lipoprotein density classes [3, 6] is compatible with the occurrence of distinct lipoprotein particles within the operationally-defined lipoproteins.

Although the discovery of apolipoproteins has added a new dimension to the heterogeneity and complexity of plasma lipoproteins, it has also provided a new criterion for characterizing and classifying individual lipoproteins. Due to their chemical uniqueness, apolipoproteins are ideal markers for identifying lipoprotein particles. To account for the chemical heterogeneity of operationally-defined lipoproteins, we proposed some 20 years ago, that lipoproteins be classified on the basis of their apolipoprotein composition [7]. According to this concept, the plasma lipoprotein system consists of a mixture of lipoprotein families or particles, each of which is characterized by a unique apolipoprotein composition. Lipoprotein families are defined as macromolecular complexes consisting of neutral lipids, phospholipids, and apolipoproteins, linked through non-convalent interactions and forming a polydisperse system of particles, heterogeneous with respect to physical properties but homogeneous with respect to their qualitative apolipoprotein composition. For example, individual particles of lipoprotein B (LP-B) family may have different hydrated densities, sizes, or lipid/protein compositions but they all contain only ApoB as their apolipoprotein constituent. Lipoprotein families which contain a single apolipoprotein are referred to as *simple* lipoproteins, and those which contain two or more apolipoproteins are called *complex* lipoproteins [2]. The nomenclature of lipoprotein families is based on the ABC nomenclature of apolipoproteins in that lipoproteins are

H. U. Klör (Ed.)
Lipoprotein Subfractions
Omega-3 Fatty Acids
© Springer-Verlag Berlin Heidelberg 1989

named according to their apolipoprotein composition. The lipoprotein family characterized by the presence of Apo B is called LP-B, and that characterized by Apo A-I and Apo A-II is called LP-A-I:A-II, etc.

The purpose of this paper is to provide a brief update of more recent studies on the chemistry and functional properties of discrete lipoprotein families or particles.

Plasma lipoproteins defined by their apolipoprotein composition can be classified into major and minor lipoproteins, each of which may contain simple and complex lipoprotein families. The ApoA- and ApoB-containing lipoprotein particles are the two major lipoprotein groups, while lipoproteins which contain only apolipoproteins C, D, E, F, G, and H are the minor lipoproteins. The Apo A- and Apo B-containing lipoproteins may be separated by immunoprecipitation or immunoaffinity chromatography of whole plasma with either polyclonal antisera to Apo B or monoclonal antibodies which bind equally to all Apo B-containing lipoproteins ("Pan B" monoclonal antibody) [8]. These two major lipoprotein groups can also be separated by affinity chromatography of whole plasma on concanavalin A. In all these procedures minor lipoproteins are also separated from Apo B-containing lipoproteins and occur together with Apo A-containing lipoproteins. They can be separated from Apo A-containing lipoproteins by further fractionation on immunosorbers with anti-Apo A-I and anti-Apo A-II sera. Fractionation of Apo A-containing lipoproteins into LP-A-I and LP-A-I:A-II lipoprotein families has been described elsewhere [9] and will not be further discussed here. Instead, this paper will be concerned with the procedures used for the fractionation of Apo B-containing lipoproteins either from whole plasma or major lipoprotein density classes including very low (VLDL, $d < 1.006$ g/ml) and low (LDL$_1$, d 1.006–1.109 g/ml and LDL$_2$, d 1.019–1.063 g/ml) density lipoproteins. The fractionation procedures used in this laboratory are either sequential immunoprecipitation or sequential immunoaffinity chromatography. As shown in Fig. 1, one aliquot of starting lipoprotein material is first precipitated by an antiserum to Apo B in order to determine the amounts of apolipoproteins C-I, C-II, C-III, and E not bound to Apo B. In the next stage, the sequential immunoprecipitation of another aliquot of the same lipoprotein starting material is initiated by precipitation of all Apo E-containing lipoproteins with an antiserum to Apo E. The amount of precipitated Apo B- and Apo E-containing lipoproteins is determined by the concentration difference between these apolipoproteins present in the starting material and in the soluble fraction remaining after the completion of precipitation with antibodies to Apo E. The precipitated lipoprotein families may consist of LP-B:C:E, LP-B:E, and LP-E. The amounts of LP-B:E and LP-E account in most subjects for less than 10% of the total Apo E. In the next step, the remaining lipoproteins are treated with an antiserum to Apo C-III; the precipitated lipoprotein families comprise LP-B:C and LP-C-III. If the soluble fraction remaining after precipitation with anti-Apo C-III contains some Apo C-I and/or Apo C-III, these lipoproteins are precipitated with corresponding anti-Apo C-I and/or anti-Apo C-II sera. If these apolipoproteins or their corresponding lipoprotein families are not present, the remaining lipoproteins consist only of LP-B particles. Application of this procedure to the fractionation of Apo B-containing lipoproteins has revealed that, in all subjects studied so far, LP-B is the major simple lipoprotein family and LP-B:C:E and LP-B:C (in both of these lipoproteins, apo C consists of all three polypeptides, i. e. C-I, C-II and C-III) are the major complex lipoprotein families. However, in fasting normolipidemic and hyper-

First Stage

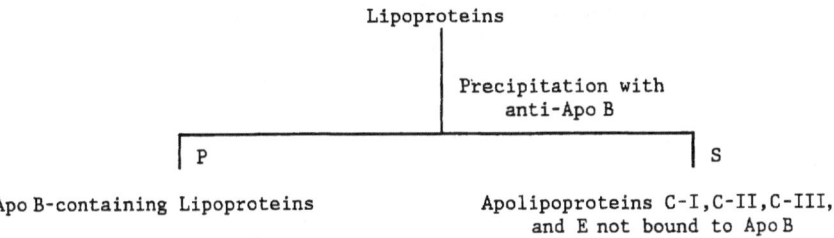

Second Stage

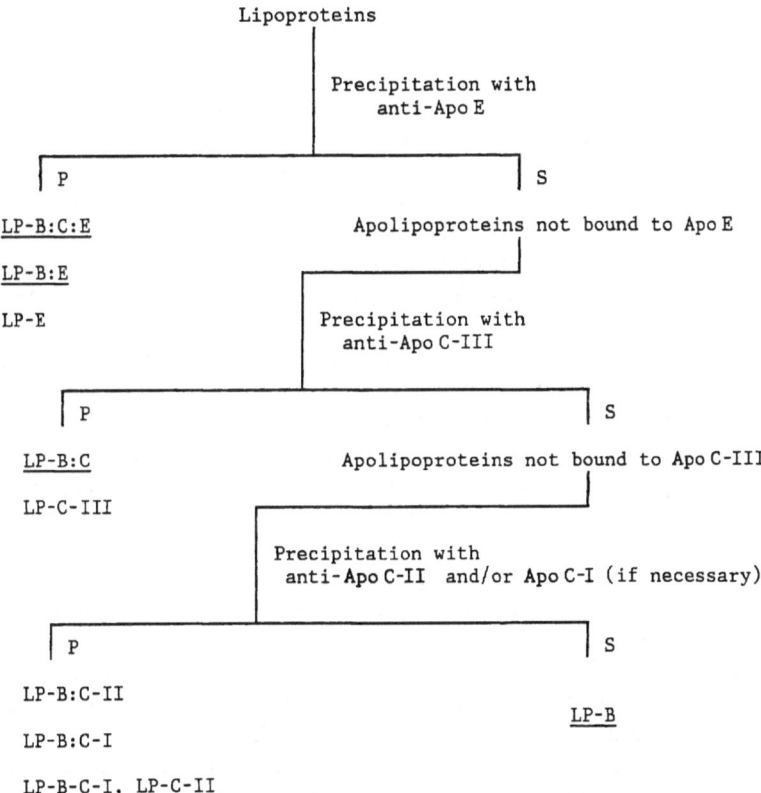

Fig. 1. Sequential immunoprecipitation of lipoproteins (VLDL, LDL$_1$, and LDL$_2$). *P*, precipitate; *S*, soluble fraction. The purpose of the first stage of the isolation procedure is to establish small quantities of apolipoproteins C-I, C-II, C-III, and E not bound to Apo B (LP-C-I, LP-C-II, LP-C-III, and LP-E) The second stage is concerned with the separation of Apo B lipoproteins which contain Apo E (LP-B:C-I:C-II:C-III:E, LP-B:E), Apo B lipoproteins which only contain Apo C (LP-B:C-I:C-II:C-III), Apo B lipoproteins which may only contain Apo C-I or Apo C-II (LP-B:C-I, LP-B:C-II), and lipoproteins which only contain Apo B (LP-B). Major lipoprotein particles are *underlined*. The same fractionation procedure can be carried out by the use of immunosorbers

cholesterolemic subjects, LP-B:E should also be considered as a major ApoB-containing lipoprotein. The identification and characterization of these lipoprotein particles is usually carried out on fractions isolated by immunoaffinity chromotography, because both the retained and unretained fractions are obtained in soluble form. The sequence of immunosorbers is the same as that of antisera used for sequential immunoprecipitation. The apolipoprotein composition of complex lipoproteins changes with increasing densities in that the relative content of Apo B increases and the relative contents of Apo C peptides and Apo E decreases. The lipid composition of Apo B-containing lipoprotein particles is characterized by a considerable degree of specificity. The LP-B particles, regardless of their density properties, contain cholesterol esters as their main neutral lipid constituent. On the other hand, LP-B:C and LP-B:C:E particles are triglyceride-rich, irrespective of their density properties.

The analysis of the apolipoprotein and lipid composition of lipoprotein particles clearly reveals their polydisperse character. This is illustrated, for example, in the case of the LP-B family isolated from whole plasma by affinity chromatography on concanavalin A and subsequent sequential immunoprecipitation of Apo B-containing lipoproteins. The fractionation of LP-B on a Sepharose-4B column results in a number of fractions, each of which is characterized by Apo B being the sole protein component. However, the measurement of neutral lipids shows that fractions of decreasing sizes have decreasing amounts of triglycerides and increasing amounts of cholesterol esters. This change in triglyceride/cholesterol ester ratios is also found in LP-B particles isolated separately from VLDL, LDL_1, and LDL_2, indicating that one of the factors contributing to the polydispersity of LP-B particles is a change in ratios of these two neutral lipids. The other important factor is the changing weight ratio of total lipid to protein.

The polydisperse character of all major Apo B-containing lipoprotein families is further demonstrated by measurement of their concentration profiles. In normolipidemic subjects, LP-B is present mainly in LDL_2 (48.0 ± 15 mg/dl) and LDL_1 (2.9 ± 2.4 mg/dl), but small amounts of LP-B (1.3 ± 0.9 mg/dl) are also detectable in VLDL. The LP-B:C:E family occurs in VLDL, LDL_1, and LDL_2 (3.4 ± 2.2, 2.1 ± 2.0, and 7.8 ± 5.9 mg/dl, respectively); all three density classes also contain relatively low concentrations of LP-B:C particles (1.7 ± 1.6, 5.0 ± 4.0, and 0.7 ± 0.4 mg/dl, respectively). The corresponding profile of patients heterozygous for familial hypercholesterolemia is characterized by high concentrations of the LP-B family in VLDL, LDL_1, and LDL_2 (2.6 ± 2.6, 8.9 ± 2.4, and 160 ± 24 mg/dl) and by a high level of LP-B:E in LDL_2 (35 ± 16 mg/dl); the concentrations of the LP-B:C family are negligent. In contrast, patients with type V hyperlipoproteinemia have relatively low concentrations of LP-B in LDL_2 (24 ± 7.2 mg/dl), but high levels of triglyceride-rich LP-B:C:E and LP-B:C in VLDL (22.3 ± 6.7 and 28.3 ± 14 mg/dl, respectively). The concentrations of lipoprotein families are expressed only in terms of their apolipoprotein levels. Preliminary studies have shown that primary and secondary hyperlipoproteinemias are characterized by specific profiles of Apo B-containing lipoprotein families.

To gain some initial information on the formation of Apo B-containing particles, we have studied recently these lipoproteins in the medium of HepG2 cells [10]. Results of this study have shown that LP-B and LP-B:E are the major lipoprotein families secreted by HepG2 cells. In contrast to their plasma counterparts, both LP-B and LP-B:E were characterized by relatively high contents of triglycerides, regardless of their hydrated densities. The possibility that the triglyceride-rich LP-B and LP-B:E particles might be the precursors of corresponding plasma LP-B:C and LP-B:C:E families remains to be tested in future experiments.

Recently, we have followed the lipoprotein lipase (LPL) catalyzed degradation of triglyceride-rich lipoproteins by measurement of Apo B-containing lipoprotein families [11]. The starting material was a VLDL preparation from normolipidemic subjects consisting mainly of LP-B:C:E particles, while human milk was used as the source of LPL. The dissociation of apolipoproteins B, C, and E was proportional to the degree of triglyceride hydrolys with LDL_2 particles as the major and LDL_1, and high density (HDL, d 1.063–1.21 gl/ml), and very high density (VHDL, $d > 1.21$ gl/ml) lipoprotein particles as the minor products of a complete in vitro lipolysis of VLDL (LP-B:C:E particles). After a 95% hydrolysis, plasma LDL_2 consisted of the 92.5% LP-B family as the main products and 2.5% LP-B:C–I:E and 5% LP-B:C families as the minor products of lipolytic degradation. These results have demonstrated that the formation of LP-B as the "ultimate" remnant of VLDL lipolysis only requires LPL as a catalyst and albumin as the fatty acid acceptor. However, under physiological circumstances, other modulating agents are necessary to prevent accumulation and regulate the interaction of phospholipid/cholesterol-rich Apo C- and Apo E-containing particles released by lipolytic degradation and dissociation of LP-B:C:E and other triglyceride-rich lipoproteins.

The rate of lipolytic degradation of triglyceride-rich lipoproteins is not only dependent upon the level of LPL, but also on the reactivity of the triglyceride-rich lipoprotein substrate with LPL. As part of our studies on the mechanism of hypertriglyceridemia in Tangier disease [12], we have examined under standardized experimental conditions the lipolysis of Tangier VLDL-triglycerides catalyzed by human milk LPL. The decreased triglyceride concentration during the time-course of lipolysis was expressed by a pseudo first-order rate constant (k_1), defined as a measure of the reactivity of triglyceride-rich lipoproteins with LPL. The k_1 values for Tangier VLDL (0.017 ± 0.002 min^{-1})were significantly lower ($p < 0.001$) than the k_1 values for control VLDL (0.036 ± 0.008 min^{-1}). The major compositional difference between VLDL from Tangier and normal subjects was a significantly higher relative content of Apo A-II in VLDL of the former than the latter subjects. To test further for a possible difference in the chemical composition of VLDL particles, the Tangier VLDL were applied onto an immunosorber with antibodies to Apo A-II, and the retained and unretained fractions were analyzed for their lipid and apolipoprotein composition. The retained fraction was characterized as a triglyceride-rich lipoprotein containing Apo A-II, B, C-I, C-II, C-III, D, and E as its protein constituents. Since additional chromatography of this lipoprotein on an immunosorber with antibodies to Apo B showed no change in the chemical composition, this newly discovered lipoprotein family was called the LP-A-II:B:C:D:E family or, in the abbreviated form, the LP-A-II:B complex. This triglyceride-rich complex accounted in Tangier disease for 80%–90% of the total VLDL on the basis of either the Apo B or triglyceride contents. The unretained fractions contained small amounts of triglyceride-rich LP-B:C:E and LP-B:C particles. Further studies have shown that this complex triglyceride-rich lipoprotein family also occurs in VLDL of normal and hyperlipoproteinemic subjects. Moreover, the LP-A-II:B complex has been detected in LDL_1 and LDL_2 of patients with Tangier disease and other dyslipoproteinemias, indicating the polydisperse character of these lipoprotein particles. The lipid composition of the LP-A-II:B complex isolated from VLDL of patients with Tangier disease or type V hyperlipoproteinemia was characterized by a high percent content of triglycerides (55%–60%) and lower contents of cholesterol esters (10%–11%), free cholesterol (5%–6%), and phospholipids (14%–16%). The lipid composition of LP-B:C:E + LP-B:C particles was very similar, if not identical, to that of the LP-A-II:B complex. However, the k_1 value of the LP-A-II:B complex (0.0148 ± 0.002 min^{-1}) was significantly lower ($p < 0.0001$) than the k_1 value of the LP-B:C:E + LP-B:C particles (0.036 ± 0.002 min^{-1}).

This finding is of considerable importance for the concept of lipoprotein families, because it demonstrates that chemically distinct lipoprotein families isolated from the same density class also have distinct biological and functional properties. An analogous finding has recently been reported for human LP-B and LP-B:E families isolated from LDL$_2$ and shown to have significantly different binding characteristics for HepG2 cell membranes [13]; LP-B had a K_d value of 69 nM and LP-B:E a value of 21 nM. Another example has been provided by recent studies [14] suggesting that LP-A-I particles, but not LP-A-I:A-II particles, from human HDL may act as promoters of cholesterol efflux from peripheral tissue and, thus, behave as distinct metabolic entities within the same lipoprotein density class. Rat HDL has been shown to contain LP-A-I, LP-E, and LP-A-I:E as the major lipoprotein families [15]. Furthermore, LP-E has been found to interact with a specific hepatic Apo E receptor, LP-A-I with a specific hepatic and renal HDL receptor, and LP-A-I:E with both Apo E and HDL receptors.

The examination of lipoprotein particle profiles of hyperlipoproteinemic patients suggests that LP-B particles of smaller sizes may be the most atherogenic among Apo B-containing lipoproteins; the relative atherogenicity of the triglyceride-rich LP-B:C:E, LP-B:E, LP-B:C, and LP-A-II:B complex remains to be established. If confirmed and extended in future studies, the initial findings of the chemical and biological specificities of lipoprotein families may provide the opportunity to assess, through determination of lipoprotein particle profiles, the extent of metabolic defect(s) and the magnitude of atherosclerotic risk, not only in superficially defined subpopulations but also in individual patients. This approach may be further strengthened if recent results indicating the specific effect of some hypolipidemic drugs on lipoprotein particles are confirmed in future studies. It has already been shown that nicotinic acid increases while probucol decreases the concentration of LP-A-I particles [16]. Studies in our laboratory have established that nicotinic acid and colestipol administered to mildly hypercholesterolemic subjects produce a significant reduction of LP-B particles (100.8 ± 16.8 to 51.6 ± 13.4 mg/dl), but no change in the levels of LP-B:C:E or LP-B:C particles [17]. On the other hand, the administration of gemfibrozil to patients with type V hyperlipoproteinemia caused significant reductions of triglyceride-rich LP-B:C:E (31.6 ± 6 to 18.1 ± 6.6 mg/dl) and LP-B:C (32 ± 14 to 19.0 ± 3.0 mg/dl) particles accompanied by a simultaneous increase in potentially atherogenic LP-B particles (32 ± 11 to 54 ± 21 mg/dl) [18]. This suggests that determination of lipoprotein particles may offer not only a new diagnostic tool but also a means for highly selective therapeutic intervention in patients with dyslipoproteinemias.

Since future testing and application of the lipoprotein family concept to clinical studies will depend to a large extent on the development of relatively simple techniques for quantification of individual lipoprotein families, it is appropriate to point out, that some progress has already been achieved in this important aspect of the chemistry and metabolism of lipoprotein particles. We have recently described an enzyme-linked differential antibody immunosorbent assay for quantitative determination of LP-A-I and LP-A-I:A-II particles [19]. To determine Apo A-I in LP-A-I:A-II particles, the microplates were coated with antibodies to Apo A-II, the nonspecific binding sites were blocked, and the plates were incubated with plasma causing the immobilization of particles containing both Apo A-I and Apo A-II. The unbound constituents of plasma were washed away, peroxidase-labeled antibody to Apo A-I was added, the plates were rewashed, peroxidase substrate added, and the resulting color was measured. Apo A-I in LP-A-I was determined by subtracting the concentration of Apo A-I linked to Apo A-II from the total plasma level of Apo A-I. This technique is, of course, applicable to measurement of any two apolipoproteins that occur in both associated (complex lipoproteins) and unassociated (simple lipoproteins) lipoprotein forms in plasma. Another promising approach is to search for monoclonal antibodies specific for an apolipoprotein epitope uniquely expressed on a chemically well-defined lipoprotein family. This is best illustrated by the recent preparation of a monoclonal antibody to human plasma Apo B that binds specifically to LP-B:E particles [13]. The possible existence and preparation of corresponding antibodies to other Apo B-containing lipoprotein particles may permit development of simple, specific enzyme-linked immunosorbent assays for their quantitative determination.

Results of these studies are providing additional evidence that distinct lipoprotein families or particles defined by their apolipoprotein composition represent the fundamental chemical and metabolic entities of the lipid transport system. The concept of lipoprotein families thus offers a new theoretical basis for describing, interpreting, and influencing processes responsible for normal as well as defective transport of triglycerides and other lipids.

Conclusions

1. The compositional and metabolic heterogeneity of operationally defined plasma lipoproteins necessitates the introduction of a classification system based on apolipoproteins as specific markers for identifying discrete lipoprotein families or particles. According to the chemical classification system, plasma lipoproteins consist of discrete simple and complex lipoproteins. Simple lipoproteins contain a single apolipoprotein, whereas complex lipoproteins contain two or more apolipoproteins.
2. The Apo A- and Apo B-containing lipoproteins are two major groups of plasma lipoproteins. Each of these two groups consists of simple and complex lipoprotein families. The major Apo A-containing lipoprotein families are LP-A-I and LP-A-I:A-II. The major Apo B-containing lipoprotein families include LP-B, LP-B:C:E, LP-B:E, LP-A-II:B:C:D:E, and LP-B:C.
3. Discrete lipoprotein families can be separated by sequential immunoprecipitation or immunoaffinity chromatography and measured by apolipoprotein quantification.

4. Major Apo B-containing lipoprotein families have specific lipid and apolipoprotein composition. They constitute polydisperse macromolecular systems, heterogeneous with respect to hydrated density, size, and lipid/protein weight ratios, but homogeneous with respect to the qualitative apolipoprotein composition.
5. The metabolism of Apo B- and Apo A-containing lipoprotein particles depends on and seems to be affected primarily by their corresponding apolipoprotein composition.
6. Hypolipidemic drugs seem to affect discrete Apo B- and Apo A-containing lipoprotein particles in a specific manner.
7. Dyslipoproteinemias are characterized by distinct profiles of Apo B-containing lipoprotein particles.

Acknowledgements. I thank my colleagues Drs. E. Koren, N. Dashti, M. Tavella, J. M. Bard, C. S. Wang, W. J. McConathy, H. U. Kloer, C. Corder, D. M. Lee, D. Weiser, Ms. C. Knight-Gibson, Ms. D. Downs, and Mr. J. D. Fesmire for their collaboration, support, and advice in gathering the experimental evidence for and further development of the lipoprotein family concept. I thank Ms. M. French for the preparation and typing of this manuscript. Parts of this study were supported by Grant HL23181 from the U.S. Public Health Service and by the resources of the Oklahoma Medical Research Foundation.

References

1. Fredrickson DS, Levy RI, Lees RS (1967) Fat transport in lipoproteins: an integrated approach to meachanism and disorders. N Engl J Med 276: 32–44, 44–103, 148–156, 215–226, 273–281
2. Alaupovic P (1982) The role of apolipoproteins in lipid transport process. La Ricerca Clin Lab 12: 3–21
3. Lippel K, Gianturco S, Fogelman A, Nestel P, Grundy SM, Fisher W, Chait A, Albers JJ, Roheim PS (1987) Lipoprotein heterogeneity workshop. Arteriosclerosis 7: 315–323
4. Alaupovic P (1984) The physiochemical and immunological heterogeneity of human plasma high-density lipoproteins. In: Miller NE, Muller GJ (eds) Clinical and metabolic aspects of high-density lipoproteins. Elsevier, Amsterdam, pp 1–45
5. Alaupovic P, Tavella M, Fesmire J (1987) Separation and identification of Apo B-containing lipoprotein particles in normolipidemic subjects and patients with hyperlipoproteinemias. Adv Exp Med Biol 210: 7–14
6. Packard CJ, Shepherd J (1985) Models and mechanisms in very low density lipoprotein metabolism. Eur J Clin Invest 15: 51–52
7. Alaupovic P (1986) Recent advances in metabolism of plasma lipoproteins: chemical aspects. Prog Biochem Pharmacol 4: 91–109
8. Alaupovic P, Koren E, McConathy WJ, Tavella M, Knight-Gibson C, Fesmire JD (1987) Immunochemical methods of isolating and characterizing Apo B-containing lipoproteins. In: Lippel K (ed) Proceedings of the Workshop on Lipoprotein Heterogeneity. National Institutes of Health, Bethesda, pp 29–43. (NIH Publication No. 87–2646)
9. Cheung M, Albers JJ (1984) Characterization of lipoprotein particles isolated by immunoaffinity chromatography. Particles containing A-I and A-II and particles containing A-I but not A-II. J Biol Chem 259: 12201–12209
10. Dashti N, Alaupovic P, Knight-Gibson C, Koren E (1987) Identification and partial characterization of discrete Apo B-containing lipoprotein particles produced by human hepatoma cell line HepG2. Biochemistry 26: 4837–4846

11. Alaupovic P, Wang CS, McConathy WJ, Weiser D, Downs D (1986). Lipolytic degradation of human very low-density lipoproteins by human milk lipoprotein lipase: the identification of lipoprotein B as the main lipoprotein degradation product. Arch Biochem Biophys 244: 226–237
12. Wang CS, Alaupovic P, Gregg RE, Brewer HB Jr (1987) Studies on the mechanism of hyper-triglyceridemia in Tangier disease. Determination of plasma lipolytic activities, k_1 values and apolipoprotein composition of the major lipoprotein density classes. Biochem Biophys Acta 920: 9–19
13. Koren E, Alaupovic P, Lee DM, Dashti N, Kloer HU, Wen G (1987) Selective isolation of human plasma low-density lipoprotein particles containing apolipoproteins B and E by use of a mono-clonal antibody to apolipoprotein B. Biochemistry 26: 2734–2746
14. Barbaras R, Puchois P, Fruchart JC, Ailhaud G (1987) Cholesterol efflux from cultured adipose cells is mediated by LPA_I particles but not by LP-A-I:A-II particles. Biochem Biophys Res Commun 142: 63–69
15. Van Tol A, van't Hooft FM, van Gent T, Dallinga-Thie GM (1987) HDL subfractions, HDL receptors and HDL turnover. Adv Exp Med Biol 210: 15–21
16. Atmeh RF, Shepherd J, Packard CJ (1983) Subpopulations of apolipoprotein A-I in human high-density lipoproteins. Their metabolic profiles and response to drug therapy. Biochim Biophys Acta 751:175–188
17. Tavella M, Alaupovic P, Blankenhorn D, Chin HP (1987) Specific effect of combined colestipol and niacin therapy on apolipoprotein B-containing particles. Arteriosclerosis 7: 494a
18. Corder C, Tavella M, Alaupovic P (1987) Effect of gemfibrozil on discrete Apo B-containing lipoproteins in patients with type V hyperlipoproteinemia. Arteriosclerosis 7: 515a
19. Koren E, Puchois P, Alaupovic P, Fesmire J, Kandoussi A, Fruchart JC (1987) Quantification of two different types of apolipoprotein A-I containing lipoprotein particles in plasma by enzyme-linked differential-antibody immunosorbent assay. Clin Chem 33: 38–43

Ultracentrifugal, Chromatographic and Electrophoretic Techniques for Lipoprotein Subfractionation

C. H. LULEY

Subfractionation of lipoproteins is a wide field which cannot be covered in detail in this presentation. Therefore, only the major principles will be described, and only representative applications will be cited. Also, since immunoaffinity is the topic of other presentations at this meeting, this most important methodology is omitted. Isoelectric focusing of lipoproteins, however, is described in some detail, since new results from our laboratory will be presented.

The basic characteristics by which lipoproteins can be separated are shown in the Table 1.

Ultracentrifugation

The historically most important criterion by which lipoproteins have been separated is that of density. The resolving power of ultracentrifugation can be increased by the use of density gradients. Considering high-density lipoproteins (HDL), Anderson and colleagues from the Donner Laboratory in Berkeley formed such a density gradient in an angle head rotor, and described two subfractions of HDL_2, which they named HDL_{2b} and HDL_{2a} [1]. HDL_{2a} is a fraction with a density between that of HDL_{2b} and that of HDL_3. However, there is substantial overlapping of these three fractions [2]. Considerably less overlapping occurs in the application of density-gradient ultracentrifugation on low-density lipoproteins (LDL). Lee described a variant of this method

Table 1. Methodology for subfractionation of lipoproteins

Method	Technical variants	Separating criterion
Ultracentrifugation	Preparative	Hydrated density
	Density gradient	
Chromatography	Gel filtration	Size
	High-pressure liquid chromatography	Size
	Affinity chromatography	Chemical composition
	Concanavalin A	of the lipoprotein surface
	Heparin sepharose	
	Hydroxylapatite	
	Chromatofocusing	Surface charge
	Immunoaffinity	Surface apolipoproteins
Electrophoresis	Gel gradient electrophoresis	Size
	Isotachophoresis	Mobility
	Isoelectric focusing	Surface charge

H. U. Klör (Ed.)
Lipoprotein Subfractions
Omega-3 Fatty Acids
© Springer-Verlag Berlin Heidelberg 1989

that allows a reproducible fractionation of LDL_2 into three subfractionations which are well separated from each other. She showed that these subfractions differed not only in density but also in lipid composition and, furthermore, between healthy subjects and patients suffering from hyperlipoproteinemias type III and type IV [3].

A variant of this procedure is the use of a zonal rotor which, due to its much larger area of the sample cavity, allows the separation of relatively large amounts of lipoproteins. Patsch et al. described three subfractions in HDL_2 and five subfractions in HDL_3 [4]. But, as in Anderson's study [2], there was considerable overlapping of fractions.

Summarizing, several statements can be made about ultracentrifugation. This technique still plays a central role for every lipidologist. However, there are inevitable disadvantages: the method is time consuming and requires an expensive apparatus and technical skill. In addition, the separation of HDL subfractions is only poor, and ultracentrifugation introduces artefacts such as loss of apolipoproteins into the lipoprotein-free infranatant. It was therefore necessary to search for alternatives.

Chromatography

Column chromatography allows subfractionation of lipoproteins by a number of criteria: size, chemical composition of the particle surface and surface charge. The first criterion, size, is utilized by size-exclusion gel chromatography. A powerful representative of this technique is High Performance Liquid Chromatography (HPLC) which has been repeatedly applied by Okazaki et al. [5]. Separating HDL from 10–30 µl plasma, they described a subfraction which belonged exclusively to HDL_2 and another subfraction which they found in HDL_3. Three more subfractions were found in both density classes. But, as with ultracentrifugation, the separation was not entirely satisfying.

Among chromatography variants which employ affinity as separating criterion, I would like to mention chromatography over hydoxylapatite. Kostner described this method first and reported eight HDL subfractions which clearly differed in terms of apolipoprotein composition, triglyceride and lipid/protein ratio [6]. The separation principle is not quite clear; it is probable that polar interactions with apolipoproteins and the polarity of surface lipids play a role.

A second affinity chromatographic procedure is based on the interaction of apolipoprotein E with heparin. This technique has been frequently employed, and two applications ought to be mentioned. Weisgraber and Mahley demonstrated the existence of a minor HDL fraction which they found in HDL_2 [7]. This subfraction contained, in contrast to the rest of HDL, apolipoprotein E. This lipoprotein may be of special interest for two reasons: (a) it binds avidly to liver receptors, and (b) it can be stimulated by cholesterol intake. Mahley speculated that this particle, which he named HDL_c, may be involved in reverse cholesterol transport [8].

Another application of heparin affinity chomatography was reported by Trezzi et al. [9]. They separated very low density lipoproteins (VLDL) into four subfractions, which they named A, B, C and D. Only fractions C and D contained measurable amounts of apolipoprotein E, and only these two subfractions interacted with human fibroblasts.

The last chromatographic procedure to be mentioned is chromatofocusing, which, like the electrophoretic techniques, separates by surface charge. Nestruck subfractionated HDL with good resolution into six fractions which differed by density, size, lipid and apolipoprotein composition [10]. She demonstrated the existence of a lipoprotein which contains apolipoprotein A-I but no apolipoprotein A-II. This particle is relatively large and "light" and is enriched with free cholesterol. This finding is an agreement with results of other investigators, including ourselves. Since several recent sets of data point to a special antiatherogenic potential of such a lipoprotein subfraction, this particle is of great interest.

Electrophoresis

The last group of subfractionating techniques described in this overview are the electrophoretic methods. Gradient gel electrophoresis is an exception among the electrophoretic techniques because it separates according to size, as does size exclusion chromatography. Blanche resolved HDL into five subfractions which she and her colleagues from the Donner laboratory assigned to the density classes HDL_{2b}, HDL_{2a} and HDL_3 [11]. The comparison of her results to those of HPLC, as mentioned above, yields only partial agreement between the characteristics described.

Mobility is the separation criterion of isotachophoresis, which offers a high power of resolution. Bon subfractionated HDL_2 into six and HDL_3 into ten bands [12]. He also showed that the obtained subfractions differed in respect to apolipoprotein and lipid composition.

The last electrophoretic technique to be mentioned is isoelectric focusing. Isoelectric focusing offers a very high power of resolution and has been a routine method in protein separation for many years. In contrast to isotachophoresis, which separates by mobility, isoelectric focusing fractionates according surface charge alone, as does chromatofocusing. Agarose is a carrier medium of special interest because it allows virtually free movement of particles which may even be as large as those of VLDL. Isoelectric focusing can be used either on an analytical or on a preparative scale. On an analytical scale, it is possible to separate LDL and HDL subfractions out of 10 µl serum [13]. When the focusing is finished, subfractions can be selectively precipitated by phosphotungstic acid/Mg^{2+} and later stained with Sudan black. An example of HDL subfractions found in different density ranges is shown in Fig. 1.

The detection of apolipoprotein contents in the bands is easily feasible by immunoprecipitation. The strips which contain the separated bands are simply incubated in monospecific antisera. Application of immunoprecipitation revealed that the majority of bands contain apolipoproteins A–I and A–II, although in differing ratios. A basic band contains the majority of apolipoprotein E while the acidic apolipoprotein C–III was found in the bands at the anodic end of the band pattern (Fig. 2) [14]. This distribution of apolipoproteins in HDL subfractions supports the assumption that the net surface charge of each particle is predominantly determined by its apolipoprotein constituents.

The characteristics of HDL subfractions as isolated by preparative isoelectric focusing correspond to those upon analytical focusing. In cooperation with Eberhard von Hodenberg (University of Heidelberg) we investigated whether isoelectric HDL

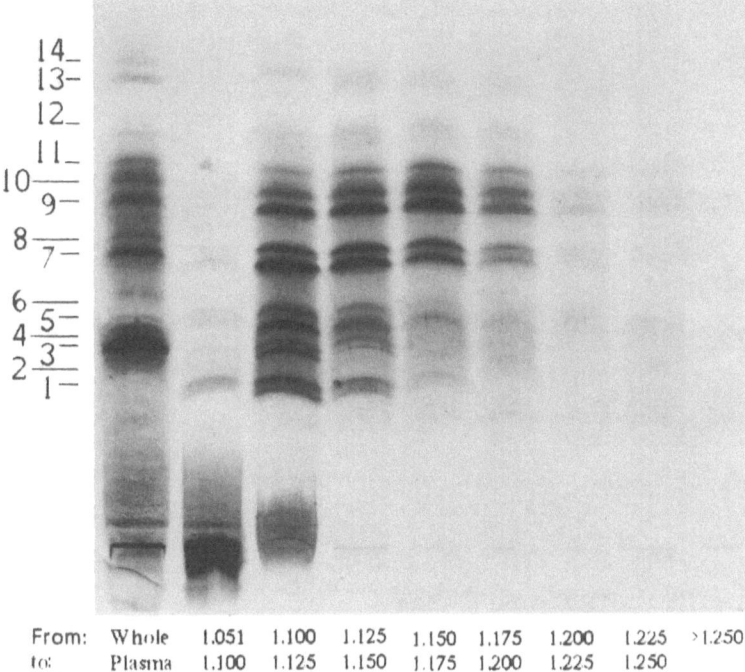

Fig. 1. Bidimensional separation of HDL subfractions. *Vertical:* Isoelectric focusing with the cathode at the bottom. *Horizontal: Left,* whole plasma, followed by density subfractions from density ranges as assigned in the graph. The bands were first precipitated in the gel and then stained with Sudan black. It is apparent that isoelectric subfractions cumulate in differing density ranges

subfractions differed in their capacity to stimulate cholesterol efflux from macrophages which had been laden with cholesterol. Preliminary data indicate that this is preferably the case for the basic subfraction which contains only apolipoprotein A–I but no apolipoprotein A–II. This subfraction is also characterized by its relatively low density, its large size and its enrichment with free cholesterol.

As mentioned above, the large pore size of agarose also allows the subfractionation of VLDL. Upon isoelectric focusing of VLDL which had been isolated by ultracentrifugation, we found three groups of bands which differ in respect to density, lipid and apolipoprotein composition. Functional differences were seen after an oral fat load and upon heparin-induced lipolysis. Acidic subfractions rich in triglycerides and apolipoprotein C–III increased after the fat load and were apparently the preferred substrate for the action of heparin-released lipases (Fig. 3).

A final consideration deals with artefacts which might be introduced by certain techniques. Lipoproteins are complex macromolecules. Some of their constituents are tightly bound to the particle while others are apparently only loosely associated. The latter appear to be easily exchangeable between lipoproteins which may be part of their physiological function. These "loose" constituents can be lost during separating procedures. An example is apolipoprotein A–IV, which is found to 90% and more

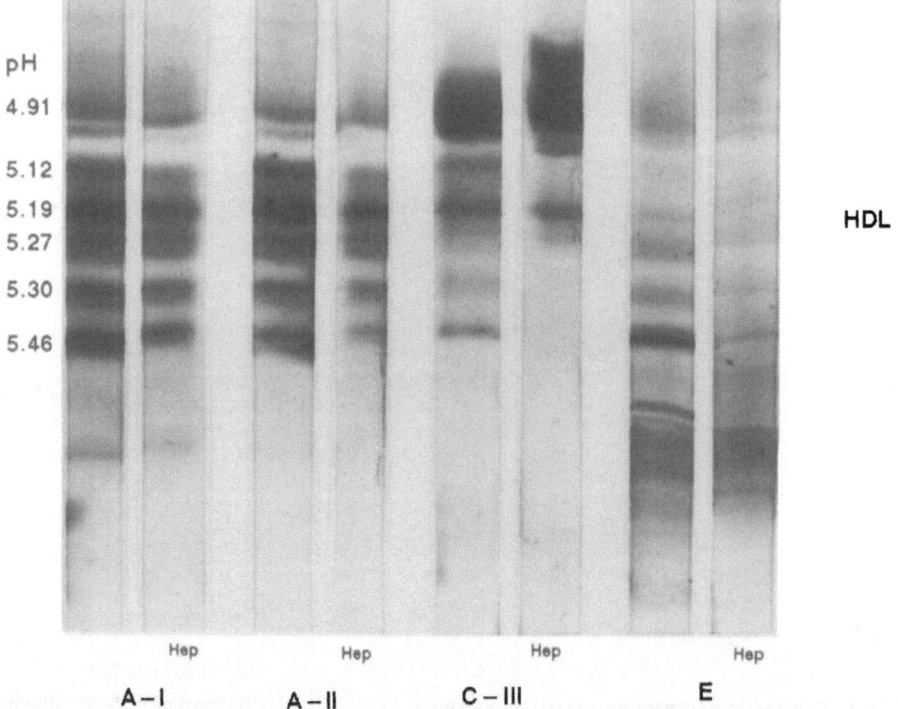

Fig. 2. Immunoprecipitation of isoelectric subfractions by monospecific antisera against apolipoproteins A–I, A–II, C–III and E. Samples were sera of a metabolically healthy donor before and after heparin-induced lipolysis *(Hep)*. The most remarkable changes in this experiment are the drastic increase of the apolipoprotein C–III-rich subfraction and the concomitant decrease of the apolipoprotein E-rich subfraction

in the lipoprotein-free infranatant upon ultracentrifugation. If agarose gel filtration is used for lipoprotein separation, a substantial amount is found in HDL. Or, when one carries out *preparative* isoelectric focusing of VLDL (which requires a focusing time of 16 h), one notices that a remarkable proportion of the C-apolipoproteins leave their lipoproteins and yield pure protein bands. This phenomenon, in contrast, did not occur in *analytical* isoelectric focusing, which takes only 1.5 h. These lipoprotein alterations, however, should not be regarded as entirely discrediting a method. In contrast, effects which are reproducibly caused by a certain technique can give additional information.

In conclusion, there are a number of techniques which allow the subfractionation of lipoproteins. However, we know that apolipoproteins are constituents which strongly determine the metabolic fate of most lipoprotein particles. Therefore, methods which subfractionate lipoproteins according to apolipoprotein composition deserve the preferred attention of any researcher who investigates functional aspects of lipoprotein subfractions.

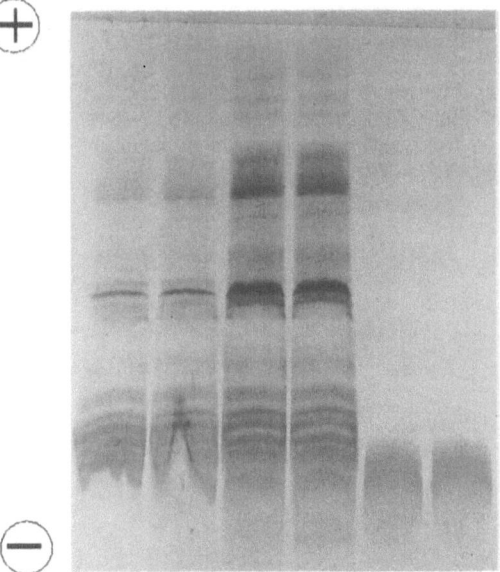

Fig. 3. Isoelectric subfractions of VLDL (duplicats). The bands which are visualized by lipid staining after precipitation by phosphotungstic acid/Mg^{2+} stem from isolated VLDL of a healthy donor before an oral fat load *(fasting)*, 2 h later *(after fat load)* and 30 min after a subsequent i.v. heparin injection *(after heparin)*

Fasting   After   After
               fat load   heparin

References

1. Anderson DW, Nichols AV, Forte TM, Lindgren FT (1977) Particle distribution of human high density lipoproteins. Biochim Biophys Acta 493: 55–68
2. Anderson DW, Nichols AV, Pan SS, Lindgren FT (1978) High density lipoprotein distribution. Resolution and determination of three major components in a normal plasma sample. Atherosclerosis 29: 161–179
3. Lee D, Downs D (1982) A quick and large-scale density gradient subfractionation method for low density lipoproteins. J Lipid Res 23: 14–27
4. Patsch W, Schonfeld G, Gotto AM jr, Patsch JR (1980) Characterization of human high density lipoproteins by zonal ultracentrifugation. J Biol Chem 255: 3178–3185
5. Okazaki M, Hagiwara N, Hara I (1982) Heterogeneity of human serum high density lipoproteins on high performance liquid chromatography. J Biochem 92: 517–524
6. Kostner GM, Holasek A (1979) The separation of human serum high density lipoproteins by hydroxylapatite column chromatography. Evidence for the presence of discrete subfractions. Biochim Biochim Acta 488: 417–431
7. Weisgraber KH, Mahley RW (1980) Subfractionation of human high density lipoproteins by heparin-sepharose affinity chromatography. J Lipid Res 21: 316–325
8. Mahley RW (1982) Atherogenic hyperlipoproteinemia. The cellular and molecular biology of plasma lipoproteins altered by dietary fat and cholesterol. In: Havel RJ (ed) The medical clinics of north america. Symposium on lipid disorders, vol 66/2. Saunders, Philadelphia, pp 375–402
9. Trezzi E, Calvi C, Roma P, Catapano AL (1983) Subfractionation of human very low density lipoproteins by heparin-sepharose affinity chromatography. J Lipid Res 24: 790–795
10. Nestruck C, Niedmann PD, Wieland H, Seidel D (1983) Chromatofocusing of human high density lipoproteins and isolation of lipoproteins A and A–I. Biochim Biophys Acta 753: 65–73
11. Blanche P, Gong EL, Forte TM, Nichols AV (1981) Characterization of human high-density lipoproteins by gradient gel electrophoresis. Biochim Biophys Acta 665: 408–419

12. Bon B, Cazzolato G, Avogaro P (1981) Preparative isotachophoresis of human plasma high density lipoproteins HDL$_2$ and HDL$_3$. J Lipid Res 22: 998–1002
13. Luley C, Watanabe H, Kloer HU (1983) Flat-bed isoelectric focusing of high density lipoproteins. J Chromatography 278: 412–417
14. Luley CH, Puchois P, Kloer HU (1984) The effect of different isolation procedures on high density lipoprotein subfractions obtained by isoelectric focusing. Clin Chim Acta 146: 185–193

Analysis of Lipoprotein Particles Using Immunoaffinity Chromatography and ELISA Techniques

J. C. Fruchart, and J. M. Bard

Apolipoproteins, supporting components of the lipoproteins, have a variety of structural and metabolic functions related to the metabolism of lipids. They are structural components for lipoprotein stability, but also co-factors for enzymes and binding ligands for cellular receptors. This has led to the use of apolipoproteins as specific markers for lipoprotein species classification. Following this concept, proposed 20 years ago by Pierre Alaupovic, one can postulate that the plasma lipoproteins consist of a mixture of particles which can be differentiated by their protein composition and contain one, two, or more apolipoproteins associated with lipids. Some of these particles are particularly atherogenic, some are less atherogenic, and others could be protective against premature atherosclerotic lesions. Thus, it is important to try to quantitate these described particles. These quantifications cause important analytical problems. Due to their specificity and elegance, the immunological procedures represent a logical choice for technical innovation in this field.

Recently, in cooperation with Eugene Koren and Pierre Alaupovic, we have developed new methodologies for what we call the molecular analysis of lipoprotein particles. This report briefly presents an immunoenzymometric assay which allows the separation of particles according to their apolipoprotein composition or according to epitope expression of one apolipoprotein on their surface.

Methods

Mapping of lipoprotein particles was obtained mainly with monoclonal antibodies. Stable mouse or rat hybridoma cell lines have been developed in our laboratory, in collaboration with others, to produce monoclonal antibodies against human apolipoproteins B, A-I, A-II, C-III, E, and (a).

Immunoenzymometric assay was performed with microtiter plates as a solid-phase antibody and enzyme-labeled antibodies as conjugate (Fig. 1). Lipoprotein particles react first with immobilized antibody 1. Unbound particles are removed by washing and excess of enzyme labeled antibody 2 is allowed to react with bound antigen. Unbound labeled antibodies are removed by washing and solid phase bound enzyme is measured. The different steps have been automatized in our laboratory.

With this assay we are able to measure in whole sera different apolipoprotein associations, such as lipoprotein particles containing A-I and A-II, containing A-I but not A-II, containing C-III and B, E and B, and (a) and B.

For example, to directly determine particles containing A-I and A-II, we coat microtiter plates with antibodies against A-II. Lipoprotein particles containing A-II

H. U. Klör (Ed.)
Lipoprotein Subfractions
Omega-3 Fatty Acids
© Springer-Verlag Berlin Heidelberg 1989

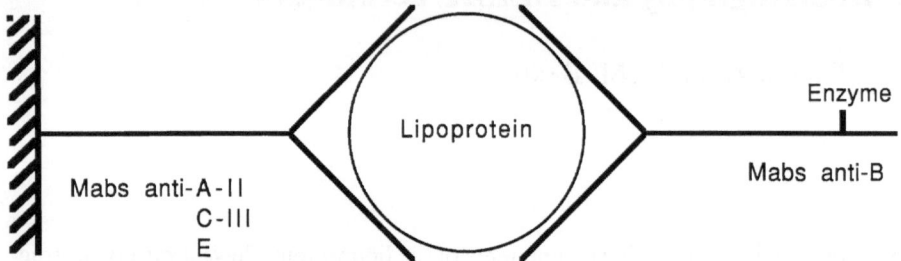

Fig. 1. Principle of the lipoprotein particle measurement

react with the antibody and we reveal the particles containing A-I and A-II with an anti A-I peroxidase label. A-I non-associated with Apo A-II is evaluated by subtracting the concentration of associated Apo A-I from the total Apo A-I concentration.

Quantification of Apo A-I Containing Particles: Clinical Applications

Apo A-I exists at least in two different types of lipoprotein particles in human plasma; more than half of the total Apo A-I is associated with Apo A-II (LpA-II:A-I), the rest occurs in lipoproteins which contain no A-II (LpA-I).

We have shown recently, in cooperation with Gérard Ailhaud's group, that these populations of particles represent two metabolically distinct pools of Apo A-I containing particles. Cholesterol efflux in cultured mouse adipocytes is mediated by LpA-I particles but not by LpA-I:A-II particles. This difference may have some clinical importance.

LpA-I and LpA-II:A-I in Coronary Artery Disease

In order to elucidate to what degree the HDL decrease observed in coronary artery disease (CAD) affects these two types of lipoprotein particles, LpA-I and LpA-I:A-II were measured in plasma from 100 male subjects with coronary artery disease as assessed by coronarography and controls. Only subjects with normal plasma lipid levels were included in the study. The results showed clearly that the decrease in Apo A-I levels for CAD subjects reflects the decrease in LpA-I particles, while LpA-II:A-I particles remain at the same level (Fig. 2). These results could be related to other studies where the decrease of HDL level in coronary artery disease has been ascribed to HDL_2 subfractions, richer in LpA-I than HDL_3.

The precise relationship between plasma A-I particle concentration and the development of atherosclerosis remains to be elucidated. Appearance of the LpA-I particle may be the reflection of the triglyceride-rich particle lipolysis in plasma. Decrease in LpA-I may be the link between atherosclerosis risk and a defective clearance of plasma triglycerides. However, our results on adipocytes suggest that a decrease in LpA-I may reflect a defect in cholesterol reverse transport.

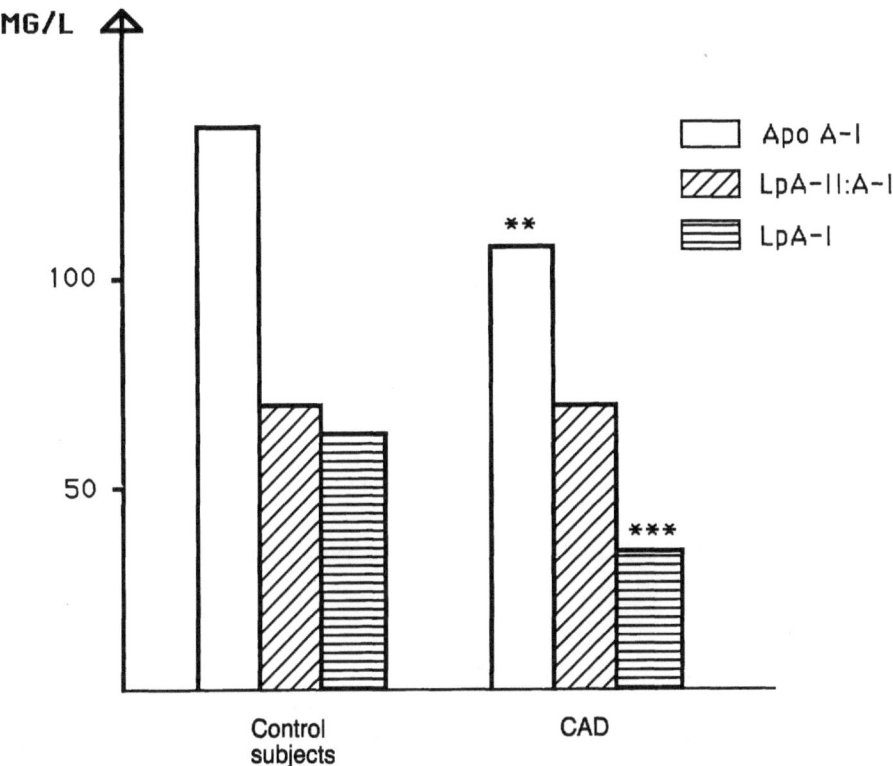

Fig. 2. Changes in LpA-I and LpA-II:A-I in coronary artery disease

LpA-I and LpA-II:A-I in Alcohol Consumption

Due to its effect on HDL cholesterol it has been suggested that moderate alcohol consumption may be protective against coronary artery disease. In order to test the effect of alcohol on Apo A-I containing particles we have measured LpA-I and LpA-I:A-II in plasma from 350 male subjects matched for age and clinical data. These subjects have been divided into five groups according to their alcohol consumption. The results confirm that alcohol consumption increases HDL cholesterol by 31%, but more remarkable is the fact that alcohol increases LpA-I:A-II particles, while it decreases LpA-I particles (Fig. 3). Thus, the increase in HDL cholesterol upon alcohol consumption reflects the increase of LpA-I:A-II, hiding the decrease in LpA-I, the lipoprotein particles probably involved in cholesterol reverse transport.

Quantification of Apo-B containing Particles: Clinical Applications

As suggested by Pierre Alaupovic, Apo B exists in different types of particles in human plasma. LpB containing only Apo B, LpB:E containing Apo B and Apo E,

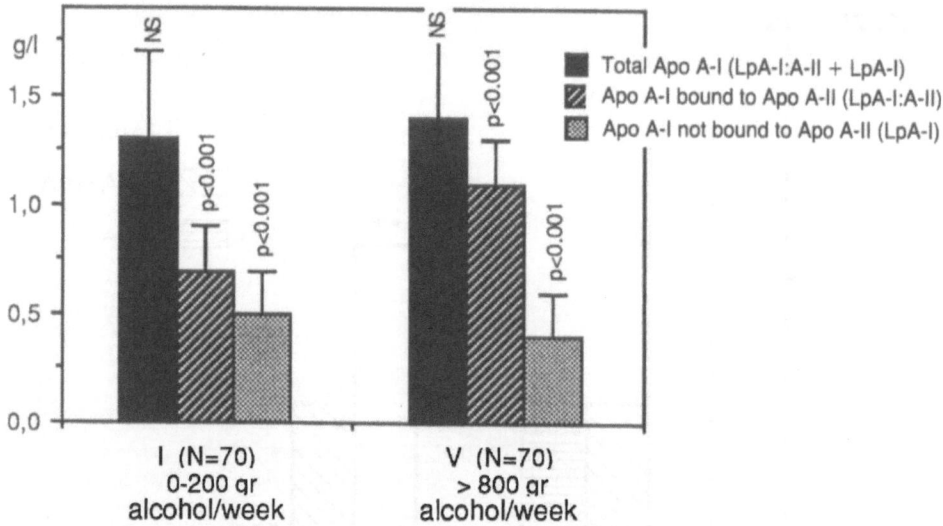

Fig. 3. Changes in LpA-I and LpA-II:A-I in relation to alcohol consumption

LpB:C-III containing Apo B and C-III, and so on. The physicochemically defined lipoproteins such as VLDL, IDL, or LDL were found to be heterogeneous with respect to this concept. A particle such as LpB, for example, may occur in any segment of the density spectrum depending on the composition and content of its lipid complement. Quantification of different Apo B containing lipoproteins is essential for better understanding of lipid transport disorders.

Lipoprotein particles containing C-III and B, E and B, can be quantitated using the assay described above. We are using in this technique a mixture of monoclonals or "pan" monoclonal, anti-C-III, anti-E and anti-(a) as first antibody, and we are using a mixture of monoclonal anti-Apo B as conjugate. In cooperation with Jean Davignon, we have recently shown that type III dyslipoproteinemia, a disorder related with accelerated atherosclerosis, is characterized by a drastically increased concentration of particles containing E and B, and to a lesser extent of particles containing C-III and B.

It is very interesting to realize that a drug like fenofibrate has various effects on the different Apo B containing particles. For example, in 50 type IIa patients, in a study done in cooperation with Philippe Douste-Blazy, we have shown that LpE:B are drastically decreased after 1 month of treatment.

In a study in collaboration with Jean Davignon, we have obtained the same type of results in 10 type III dyslipoproteinemic patients. After 1 month of treatment, fenofibrate dramatically decreased LpE:B particles (Fig. 4). Concerning these effects, three hypotheses can be entertained. First, a concomitant decrease of Apo B, Apo E, and Apo C-III could lead to less association between these apolipoproteins. Second, fenofibrate could induce the B, E receptor specific pathway for the catabolism of lipoproteins containing particularly Apo B and Apo E. Third, these lipoproteins could be submitted to a higher lipolysis rate.

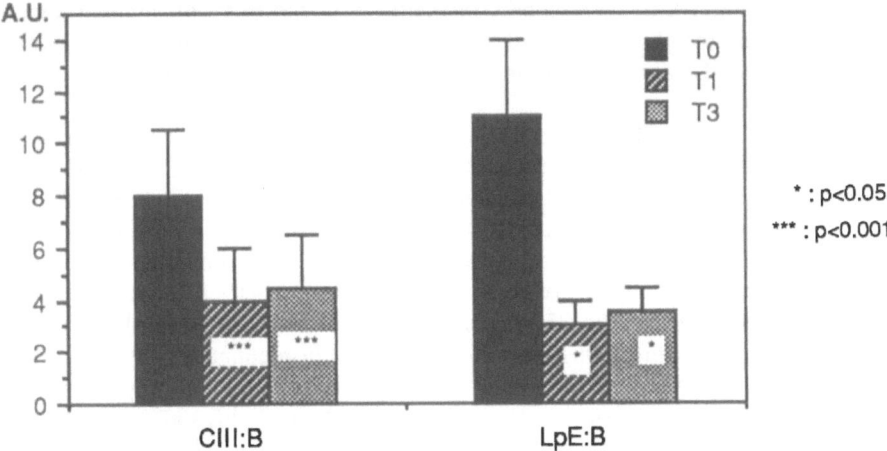

Fig. 4. Changes in lipoprotein particles of type III patients under fenofibrate therapy

Another example is given by the study of 50 patients with renal disease leading to hemodialysis. As already outlined by Pierre Alaupovic, we have found a very significant increase in LpC-III:B and a highly significant increase in particles containing (a) and B (Lp(a):B) in patients on hemodialysis. These abnormalities may accelerate the development of atherosclerosis in these patients.

Separation of Apo-B Containing Particles According to the Epitope Expression of One Apolipoprotein in Their Surface

Monoclonal antibodies can be used as first antibody in our immunoenzymometric assay. As any single epitope of an apolipoprotein may be more or less exposed depending on which particle one is examining, monoclonal antibodies can separate lipoproteins that may be similar by physicochemical criteria.

To evaluate the potential correlation between specific epitopes on B lipoprotein subpopulations and predisposition to coronary artery disease, recently we have quantitated lipoprotein particles recognized by three well-characterized monoclonal antibodies in normal and CAD patients.

These antibodies have been produced from mice at the Research Center Clin-Midy and studied in cooperation with Professor Polonovski's group. Briefly, they are called BL3, BL5, BL7. BL3 has a high affinity for LDL and VLDL, while BL5 and BL7 have a higher affinity for LDL than for VLDL. We have tested patients with normal coronaries, patients with abnormal coronaries, and other male volunteers using this technique. Patients with coronary artery disease have a significant increase in all B particles compared with controls. Using discriminant analysis, we have shown that particles recognized by monoclonal antibodies and particularly by one of them, BL3, contribute to better discrimination of the studied groups. Thus, it is possible that some subpopulation of Apo B containing apolipoproteins are more abundant in atherosclerotic patients and could be distinguished immunochemically from others.

We also studied LpB immunoheterogeneity in 24 subjects with familial hypercholesterolemia and observed that particles recognized by monoclonal antibodies and particularly by BL3 are relatively more abundant in hypercholesterolemic patients than in controls.

In order to examine the effects of drugs like fenofibrate on the plasma concentration of the various lipoproteins, we conducted in cooperation with Philippe Douste-Blazy and Pierre Drouin, a double-blind randomized placebo-control study in 40 type II_A patients. Of particular interest is the fact that the drug induced various effects on particles recognized by different monoclonal antibodies. After 1 month of treatment, the most important decreasing effect was obtained on particles recognized by BL3, while particles recognized by BL5 are not decreased. It is well established that the incidence of atherosclerotic vascular disease is higher in adequately controlled type I diabetics than in the general population. It is also well known that proper glycemic control in these patients results in normalization of plasma lipids and apolipoprotein profiles. In fact, recently we have shown in 80 patients compared with controls that diabetic lipoprotein particles have a characteristic pattern. We observed that diabetics have a significant decrease in particles recognized by BL3 and a significant increase in particles recognized by BL5. Since we have found that diabetic patients have a decrease in the ratio, LpB phospholipid/LpB cholesterol, this could be related to a modified content of LpB particles in lipids.

Conclusion

The results presented here substantiate the usefulness of the study of lipoprotein particles defined by their apolipoprotein composition for future clinical, pharmacological, and epidemiological studies. This approach might also improve our understanding of lipoprotein metabolism and different physiopathological states.

Lipoprotein Association and Function of Apolipoprotein A-IV

A. Steinmetz, and H. Kaffarnik

Introduction

Ever since it was first mentioned in the literature [35], apolipoprotein (Apo) A-IV has been of particular interest, both in terms of its appearance in plasma and in interpretation of its physiologic relevance compared with that of other apolipoproteins. Although reported to occur mainly free in human plasma unassociated with lipoproteins, its amphiphilic character as an apoprotein was demonstrated very early [2, 36]. It was also shown that the gut and the liver are the main organs synthesizing Apo A-IV [43], and recent data from messenger ribonucleic acid (mRNA) studies indicate that in the human adult the gut might be the most important source of synthesis of this apoprotein [11], indicating a major role in intestinal lipoprotein metabolism. Up to now Apo A-IV has not been shown conclusivly to have a specific function, but evidence for its having various functions, including in intestinal lipoprotein metabolism and reverse cholesterol transport, is accumulating. This contribution deals with the lipid-binding properties of Apo A-IV and current views concerning its function in lipid metabolism.

Lipid Binding Properties

Although apoprotein A-IV exhibits the properties of an apolipoprotein [2], and recent data on its sequence [11, 12, 21] have shown that it contains 14.5 tandemly repeated docosapeptides that possess the potential to form amphipathic α-helices [11], it is mainly found unassociated with lipoproteins in human plasma [4, 18, 19, 36]. The Apo A-IV fraction in the lipoprotein-free plasma compartment is still able to bind lipids, as shown by Weinberg and Scanu [37], who were able to reassociate Apo A-IV from the $d = 1.21$ g/ml infranate to a phospholipid-triglyceride emulsion. After reassociation Apo A-IV could be isolated by flotation in chylomicron-like particles upon ultracentrifugation.

After synthesis in enterocytes (increasing in response to intestinal lipid absorption) Apo A-IV is secreted as a major apoprotein component of chylomicrons and is transported in the lymph ducts (for review see [17]). Upon entry into the blood plasma compartment, it rapidly dissociates from chylomicrons and is found in the lipoprotein-free plasma fraction. Weinberg und Spector [38] showed a difference in isoform distribution between lymph and plasma Apo A-IV. Treatment of lymph Apo A-IV with neuraminidase could not mimic the isopeptide change seen upon entry into the plasma compartment [38]. The authors showed that changes in Apo A-IV isoform

H. U. Klör (Ed.)
Lipoprotein Subfractions
Omega-3 Fatty Acids
© Springer-Verlag Berlin Heidelberg 1989

distribution are associated with an alteration in lipid binding properties to the surface of model chylomicrons. Physicochemical data from Weinberg and Spector [39, 40], showed that human plasma Apo A-IV appeared to be marginally stable in aqueous solution and to have lipid binding properties sensitive to the environment, and data were consistent with Apo A-IV circulating in plasma mainly self-associated as a homodimer.

Several pools of plasma Apo A-IV were postulated, mainly from distribution and metabolic studies including tracer kinetics [15, 24]. The pools consist of Apo A-IV associated with lipoproteins of very low density, namely chylomicrons, with HDL, and in the lipoprotein-free fraction, and evidence was obtained for compartmentaliza-tion of Apo A-IV in HDL and the lipoprotein-free fraction [15].

The possible mechanism of Apo A-IV displacement from the surface of chylomi-crons upon entry into the plasma was studied in an in vitro model by Weinberg and Spector [41]. They used Apo A-IV associated with a phospholipid-triglyceride emul-sion for displacement studies. When these chylomicron-like particles were incubated with HDL, they found a displacement of Apo A-IV from these particles, mainly by Apo C-III. Thus, one of the mechanisms responsible for the dissociation of Apo A-IV from chylomicrons upon entry into the plasma compartment could be a displacement by other circulating apoproteins that have a higher affinity for chylomicrons (or their remnants after attack by lipoprotein lipase). In contrast to Apo A-IV, which decays and is later mostly found in the lipoprotein-free plasma compartment, the other major chylomicron apoprotein, A-I, reassociates with HDL, as shown by tracer kinetic studies [20, 29]. It thus remains puzzling why the bulk of Apo A-IV, despite its apoprotein structure, does not reassociate with lipoproteins. In addition, lymph and plasma Apo A-IV have similar α-helical contents and properties in solution [10]. This seems to be an unexplained phenomenon since we were able to show that apoprotein A-IV, isolated either from chylomicrons or from lipoprotein-free plasma, recombines with lipids to form stable complexes [34].

We incorporated isolated Apo A-IV into complexes with dimyristoyl-phosphatidyl-choline (DMPC) and cholesterol by the cholate dialysis procedure at a molar ratio of 150 : 1 (PC : protein). When these complexes were chromatographed on a gel filtration column (Sepharose 6 B), they eluted as a homogeneous peak. As shown in Fig. 1, these particles were slightly larger than apoprotein A-I particles produced by the same procedure and with the same molar ratios of phospholipid : protein and cholesterol contents. Interestingly, there was no apoprotein A-IV found "free", i. e., not associated with lipids, in these preparations. Furthermore, when these complexes were subjected to density gradient ultracentrifugation following the procedure of Redgrave et al. [26], they remained stable without dissocation of apoprotein. Figure 2 shows the results of such an experiment, where Apo A-IV-DMPC particles were ultracentrifuged and compared to complexes containing Apo A-I. Both complex preparations floated at a density of about 1.1 g/ml, similar to densities reported for other apoprotein/lipid complexes. As Apo A-IV is a polymorphic protein, we isolated one frequent polymorphic from Apo A-IV-2 [23] and studied its lipid-binding proper-ties. Both the obvious wild type, Apo A-IV-1, and the variant, Apo A-IV-2, exhibit the same apparent molecular weight upon SDS polyacrylamide gel eletrophoresis (see Fig. 3) and also form stable complexes with DMPC. Figure 4 shows a density gradient ultracentrifugation of Apo A-IV-1- and Apo A-IV-2-DMPC complexes. Similarly,

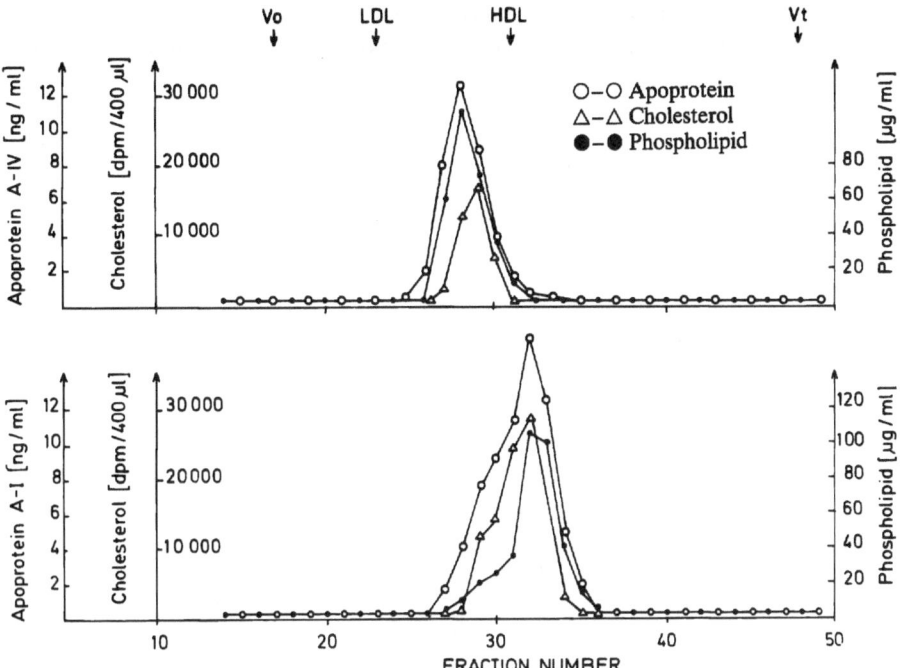

Fig. 1. Gel filtration chromatography of Apo A-IV and Apo A-I/DMPC/cholesterol complexes prepared by the cholate dialysis procedure. Apo A-IV was isolated from lipoprotein-deficient serum and Apo A-I from HDL. Note that Apo A-IV completely associates with lipids and elutes at a volume slightly less than Apo A-I/lipid complexes

Apo A-IV isolated from a rat plasma fraction of $d > 1.21$ g/ml also reassociated with DMPC to form stable complexes [27].

Thus, other factors presumably in the plasma environment and probably also differences in the phospholipid compositions of lipoproteins and the presence of other apolipoproteins may play a major role in directing Apo A-IV into the lipoprotein-free plasma compartment.

Function of Apo A-IV

Intestinal Lipoprotein Metabolism

Quite an array of studies suggested that one function of Apo A-IV is in the formation and secretion of chylomicrons (for review see [17]). Recent data show that the production of Apo A-IV mRNA in rat enterocytes is stimulated by acute triglyceride feeding [1, 16, 25]. Studies in humans also argue for a stimulation of intestinal Apo A-IV synthesis by triglyceride feeding [4, 18, 32]. Intestinal Apo A-IV production obviously contributes to the postprandial elevation of plasma Apo A-IV levels seen in man [4, 18] and rats [7]. As no patient has yet been found who could not produce Apo A-IV (Apo A-IV deficient), we do not know how such a deficiency would affect intestinal lipoprotein formation.

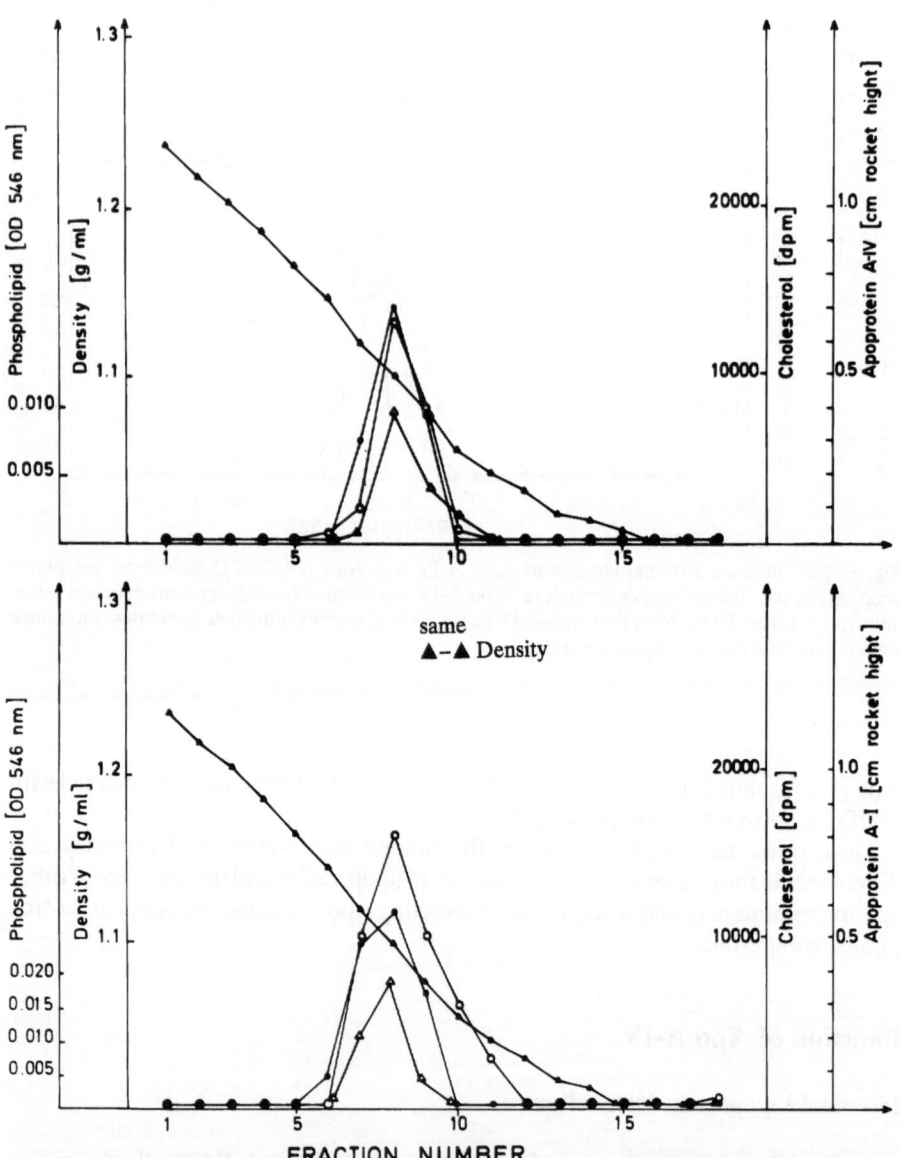

Fig. 2. Density gradient ultracentrifugation of Apo A-IV- and Apo A-I/DMPC-cholesterol complexes. The complexes were prepared as outlined in Fig. 1. After density gradient ultracentrifugation [26], tubes were punctured from the bottom and 0.5-ml fractions were collected. The density of apolipoprotein/lipid complexes of both Apo A-IV and Apo A-I was determined as 1.1 g/ml. They remained stable upon ultracentrifugation. *Upper panel,* results for Apo A-IV; *lower panel,* for Apo A-I

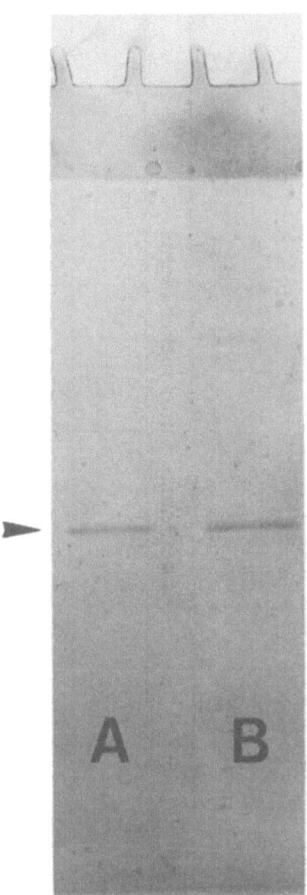

Fig. 3. Sodium docecylsulfate polyacrylamide gel electrophosesis of Apo A-IV polymorphic forms. Apo A-IV-1 (wild type) and Apo A-IV-2 (variant) were isolated from lipoprotein-deficient serum as described by Weinberg and Scanu [37] and modified by Steinmetz and Utermann [34]. *Left lane* shows Apo A-IV-1, *right lane* Apo A-IV-2. Both apoproteins exhibit similar apparent molecular weight in this system

Reverse Cholesterol Transport

Several mechanisms of lipid metabolism have now been linked to reverse cholesterol transport, including the lipid transfer protein (LTP) reaction, the activity of lecithin:cholesterol acyltransferase (LCAT), and the removal of cholesterol from cells (cholesterol efflux). Reports in the literature link the function of Apo A-IV to these three processes. Weinberg and Spector [42] concluded from their experiments that Apo A-IV could function as, or in concert with, a lipid transfer factor. Lagrost et al. [22] showed that a small HDL-like particle was formed in human serum in vitro upon incubation with partially purified lipid transfer protein and Apo A-IV. Furthermore, Apo A-IV was shown to activate LCAT in vitro [5, 33, 34], and the plasma distribution of Apo A-IV appeared to be dependent on the LCAT reaction in rats [6] and humans [3]. Evidence also exists to link Apo A-IV to the LCAT reaction in vivo. This is supported by the observation that plasma of Apo A-I-deficient patients [13] contains normal amounts of cholesteryl ester.

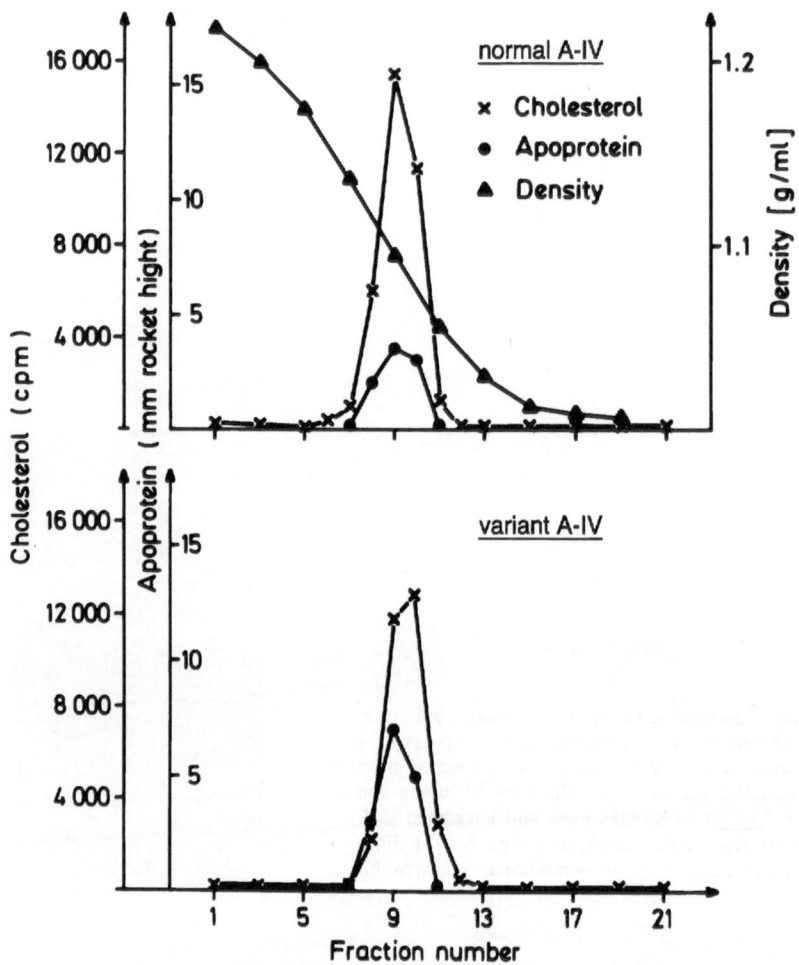

Fig. 4. Density gradient ultracentrifugation of apolipoprotein A-IV/phospholipid/cholesterol complexes. Apo A-IV-1 (wild type) and Apo A-IV-2 (variant) /lipid complexes were prepared by the dialysis detergent procedure and subjected to density-gradient ultracentrifugation as outlined in Fig. 2. Note that the variant Apo A-IV-2 peptide forms stable complexes with lipids as the wild type, Apo A-IV-1

The promotion of cholesterol efflux from cells could be the first step in reverse cholesterol transport. In their experiments using cholesterol-loaded human skin fibroblasts, Stein and colleagues [31] showed a significant enhancement of cholesterol efflux by Apo A-IV/phospholipid complexes. It is not yet fully understood how apoproteins promote cellular cholesterol efflux. Evidence is accumulating that a specific receptor-mediated process is involved. Thus far, it has been shown that Apo A-IV binds to cells and membrane preparations from different species. Ghiselli et al. [14] concluded from their experiments that rat Apo A-IV/DMPC complexes bound specifically in a saturable manner to rat liver membranes. Along the same line, Dvorin and colleagues [9] showed that rat Apo A-IV was one of the ligands responsible for the binding of rat HDL to rat hepatocytes. This binding site differs from Apo E-dependent receptors (Apo B, E and chylomicron remnant receptors). Recently, Savion and colleagues [28] demonstrated that Apo A-I and A-IV, present in human lipoprotein-deficient serum, were able to displace radiolabeled HDL bound to bovine aortic endothelial cells. The evidence for a role of Apo A-IV in reverse cholesterol transport is further strengthened by the observation that Apo A-IV is a major apoprotein component of peripheral lymph and interstitial fluid [6, 8, 30]. At present there seems to be no evidence linking the various possible functions of apoprotein A-IV to a common role in lipid metabolism, and further experiments are needed to unravel the secrets surrounding this unusual apoprotein.

Acknowledgement. The work of the author cited here was supported by a grant from the Deutsche Forschungsgemeinschaft to A. S.

References

1. Apfelbaum TF, Davidson NO, Glickman RM (1987) Apolipoprotein A-IV synthesis in rat intestine: regulation by dietary triglyceride. Am J Physiol: 252: G662–G666
2. Beisiegel U, Utermann G (1979) An apolipoprotein homolog of rat apolipoprotein A-IV in human plasma. Isolation and partial characterization. Eur J Biochem 93: 601–608
3. Bisgaier CL, Sachdev OP, Lee ES, Williams KJ, Blum CB, Glickman RM (1987) Effect of lecithin: cholesterol acyltransferase on distribution of apolipoprotein A-IV among lipoproteins of human plasma. J Lipid Res 28: 693–703
4. Bisgaier CL, Sachdev OP, Megna L, Glickman RM (1985) Distribution of apolipoprotein A-IV in human plasma. J Lipid Res 26: 11–25
5. Chen CH, Albers JJ (1985) Activation of lecithin: cholesterol acyltransferase by apolipoproteins E-2, E-3 and A-IV isolated from human plasma. Biochim Biophys Acta 836: 279–285
6. DeLamatre JG, Hoffmeier CA, Lacko AG, Roheim PS (1983) Distribution of apoliprotein A-IV between the lipoprotein and the lipoprotein-free fractions of rat plasma: possible role of lecithin: cholesterol acyltransferase. J Lipid Res 24: 1578–1585
7. DeLamatre JG, Roheim PS (1983) The response of apolipoprotein A-V to cholesterol feeding in rats. Biochim. Biophys. Acta 751: 210–217
8. Dory L, Boquet LM, Hamilton RL, Sloop CH, Roheim PS (1985) Heterogeneity of dog interstitial fluid (peripheral lymph) high density lipoproteins: implications for a role in reverse cholesterol transport. J Lipid Res 26: 519–527
9. Dvorin E, Gorder NL, Benson DM, Gotto AM Jr (1986) Apolipoprotein A-IV. A determinant for binding and uptake of high density lipoproteins by rat hepatocytes. J Biol Chem 261: 15714–15718
10. Dvorin E, Mantulin WW, Rhode MF, Gotto AM Jr, Pownall HJ, Sherill BC (1985) Conformational properties of human and rat apolipoprotein A-IV. J Lipid Res 26: 38–46
11. Elshourbagy NA, Walker DW, Boguski MS, Gordon JI, Taylor JM (1986) The nucleotide and derived amino acid sequence of human apolipoprotein A-IV mRNA and the close linkage of its gene to the genes of apolipoproteins A-I and C-III. J Biol Chem 261: 1998–2002
12. Elshourbagy NA, Walker DW, Paik YK, Boguski MS, Freeman M, Gordon JI, Taylor JM (1987) Structure and expression of the human apolipoprotein A-IV gene. J Biol Chem 262: 7973–7981
13. Forte TM, Nichols AV, Krauss RM, Norum RA (1984) Familial apolipoprotein A-I and apolipoprotein C-III deficiency. Subclass distribution, composition, and morphology of lipoproteins in a disorder associated with premature atherosclerosis. J Clin Invest 74: 1601–1613
14. Ghiselli G, Crump WL, Gotto AM Jr (1986) Binding of Apo A-IV – phospholipid complexes to plasma membranes of rat liver. Biochem Biophys Res Commun 139: 122–128

15. Ghiselli G, Krishnan S, Beigel Y, Gotto AM Jr (1986) Plasma metabolism of apolipoprotein A-IV in humans. J Lipid Res 27: 813–827
16. Gordon JI, Smith DP, Alpers DH, Strauss AW (1982) Cloning of complementary deoxyribonucleic acid encoding a portion of rat intestinal preapolipoprotein A-IV messenger ribonucleic acid. Biochemistry 21: 5424–5431
17. Green PHR, Glickman RM (1981) Intestinal lipoprotein metabolism. J Lipid Res 22: 1153–1173
18. Green PHR, Glickman RM, Riley JW, Quintet E (1980) Human apolipoprotein A-IV. Intestinal origin and distribution in plasma. J Clin Invest 65: 911–919
19. Green PHR, Glickman RM, Saudek CO, Blum CB, Tall AR (1979) Human intestinal lipoproteins: studies in chyluric subjects. J Clin Invest 84: 233–242
20. Imaizumi K, Fainaru M, Havel RJ (1978) Composition of proteins of mesenteric lymph chylomicrons in the rat and alterations produced upon exposure of chylomicrons to blood serum and serum proteins. J Lipid Res 19: 712–722
21. Karathanasis SK, Yunis I, Zannis VI (1986) Structure, evolution, and tissue-specific synthesis of human apolipoprotein A-IV. Biochemistry 25: 3962–3970
22. Lagrost L, Gambert P, Bastivas S, Athias A, Lallemant C (1987) Role of human apolipoprotein A-IV in promoting the formation of very small lipoprotein particles. 2nd European Workshop on Lipid Metabolism, Munich, November 6–7 52 (Abstract)
23. Menzel HJ, Kövary PM, Assmann G (1982) Apolipoprotein A-IV polymorphism in man. Hum Genet 62: 349–352
24. Ohta T, Fidge NH, Nestel PJ (1985) Studies on the in vivo and in vitro distribution of apolipoprotein A-IV in human plasma and lymph. J Clin Invest 76: 1252–1260
25. Pessah M, Salvat C, Amit N, Infante R (1985) Isolation and characterization of rat intestinal polyribosomes and mRNA during absorption of fat. Increased translation in vitro of Apo A-IV. Biochem Biophys Res Commun 126: 373–381
26. Redgrave TG, Robert DC, West CE (1975) Separation of plasma lipoproteins by density-gradient ultracentrifugation. Anal Biochem 65: 42–49
27. Rifici VA, Eder HA, Swaney JB (1985) Isolation and lipid-binding properties of rat apolipoprotein A-IV. Biochim Biophys Acta 834: 205–214
28. Savion N, Gamliel A, Tauber JP, Gospodarowicz, D (1987) Free apolipoproteins A-I and A-IV present in human plasma displace high-density lipoprotein on cultured bovine aortic endothelial cells. Eur J Biochem 164: 435–443
29. Schaefer EJ, Jenkins LJ, Brewer HB Jr (1978) Human chylomicron apolipoprotein metabolism Biochem Biophys Res Commun 80: 405–412
30. Sloop CH, Dory L, Roheim PS (1987) Interstitial fluid lipoproteins. J Lipid Res 228: 225–237
31. Stein O, Stein Y, Lefevre M, Roheim PS (1986) The role of apolipoprotein A-IV in reverse cholesterol transport studied with cultured cells and liposomes derived from an ether analog of phosphatidylcholine. Biochim Biophys Acta 878: 7–13
32. Steinmetz A, Czekelius P, Thiemann E, Motzny S, Kaffarnik H (1988) Changes of apolipoprotein A-IV in the human neonate: evidence for different inductions of apolipoproteins A-IV and A-I in the postpartum period. Atherosclerosis 69: 21–27
33. Steinmetz A, Kaffarnik H, Utermann G (1985) Activation of phosphatidylcholine-sterol acyltransferase by human apolipoprotein E isoforms. Eur J Biochem 152: 747–751
34. Steinmetz A, Utermann G (1985) Activation of lecithin: cholesterol acyltransferase by human apolipoprotein A-IV. J Biol Chem 260: 2258–2264
35. Swaney JB, Reese H, Eder HA (1974) Polypeptide composition of rat high density lipoprotein: characterization by SDS-gel electrophoresis. Biochem Biophys Res Commun 59: 513–519
36. Utermann G, Beisiegel U (1979) Apolipoprotein A-IV: a protein occuring in human mesenteric lymph chylomicrons and free in plasma. Isolation and quantification. Eur J Biochem 99: 333–343
37. Weinberg RB, Scanu AM (1983) Isolation and characterization of human apolipoprotein A-IV from lipoprotein-depleted serum. J Lipid Res 24: 52–59
38. Weinberg RB, Spector MS (1985) Isoform heterogeneity and lipid affinity of human lymph and plasma apolipoprotein A-IV. Biochem Biophys Res Commun 129: 576–583
39. Weinberg RB, Spector MS (1985) Structural properties and lipid binding of human apolipoprotein A-IV. J Biol Chem 260: 4914–4921
40. Weinberg RB, Spector MS (1985) The self-association of human apolipoprotein A-IV. Evidence for an in vivo circulating dimeric form. J Biol Chem 260: 14279–14286

41. Weinberg RB, Spector MS (1985) Human apolipoprotein A-IV: displacement from the surface of triglyceride-rich particles by HDL_2-associated C-apoproteins. J Lipid Res 26: 26–37
42. Weinberg RB, Spector MS (1986) Lipoprotein affinity of human apolipoprotein A-IV during cholesterol esterification. Biochem Biophys Res Commun 135: 756–763
43. Wu AL, Windmüller HG (1979) Relative contributions by liver and intestine to individual plasma apolipoproteins in the rat. J Biol Chem 254: 7316–7322

LP-X and Other Abnormal Lipoprotein Particles in Secondary Dyslipoproteinemia

H. WIELAND

An abnormal lipoprotein was once defined according to the following criteria: inappropritate lipid composition of density class (by this way the beta-VLDL of type III hyperlipoproteinemia was detected) or unusual protein content of density class (LP (a)). Both criteria led to the detection of lipoprotein X (LP-X).

Now, 15 years later, we have a more sophisticated way of defining an abnormal lipoprotein. It is either an unphysiological particle not usually occurring in the blood or a modified particle, which, because of a long residence time, has been altered by ongoing metabolic processes. In addition, it may reflect a dysequilibrium of the plasma lipoprotein system. Most abnormal lipoproteins are a consequence of such a dysequilibrium in secondary dyslipoproteinemias.

The classical abnormal lipoprotein is beta-VLDL. The E-II homozygosity leads to an impaired interaction with both the remnant receptor and the B:E receptor with a consequent slow catabolism of VLDL- or chylomicron remnants. Ongoing transfer of cholesteryl esters to these large particles causes an unusual lipid composition of the thus modified particles and a consequent dysequilibrium of the lipoprotein system. Large amounts of Apo-E are found in VLDL, and the concentration of LDL or better LP-B is markedly decreased.

A rather common abnormality is the so-called hyperapobetalipoproteinemia, according to the criteria of Sniderman (LDL cholesterol below 200 mg/dl, but LDL-Apo-B higher than 125 mg/dl). This condition is found in 34% of patients selected for coronary angiography and found to have a stenosis narrowing at least 50% of one artery. It is undefined in terms of lipoprotein particles. Is it an increase of LP-B:LP-C particles in the LDL class or is it really a lipoprotein of abnormal composition in the sense that the core is rich in triglycerides instead of cholesteryl esters?

To our surprise, hyperapobetalipoproteinemia is found more commonly in people who do not have coronary heart disease. With our technique (solubilization of LDL precipitated with heparin at pH 5.12, determination of cholesterol, and immunoassay of Apo-B by kinetic nephelometry) we find hyperapobetalipoproteinemia not to be a risk factor.

Several conditions can lead to the formation of abnormal plasma lipoproteins. A well-known possibility is the nephrotic syndrome where we have a plasmatic activator of HMG-CoA reductase and in addition difficulties in excreting mevalonic acid. This leads to a strongly increased production of cholesterol and lipoproteins. In renal insufficiency there is an increase of LP-B:LP-C-III particles in the LDL density range. This means a dysequilibrium.

It is reported in the literature, that in diabetes mellitus there is, in view of the amount of cholesterol, an unexpectedly low concentration of Apo-B in the LDL class,

H. U. Klör (Ed.)
Lipoprotein Subfractions
Omega-3 Fatty Acids
© Springer-Verlag Berlin Heidelberg 1989

i. e., a hypoapobetalipoproteinemia. This is probably due to significant amounts of lipoprotein-E carrying cholesterol but not Apo-B.

In hypothyroidism we have the down-regulation of B:E receptors, in hyperthyroidism the HDL class contains cholesterol-poor Apo-B-containing lipoproteins of electrophoretic beta-mobility.

Another source of abnormal lipoproteins lies in environmental influences like alcohol and steroids. These conditions predominantly influence the catabolism of different subpopulations of high-density lipoproteins.

Chronic renal insufficiency is treated by different forms of hemodialysis, hemofiltration, or continuous ambulatory peritoneal dialysis (CAPD). All patients have low HDL levels but show a relative increase in A-I. This condition may be called hyperapoalphalipoproteinemia.

Lipoprotein concentrations in diabetic subjects are not strikingly different from normals. LDL and VLDL are somewhat higher, HDL slightly lower. The reason for the statistical significance of the difference in our data is the large number of individuals in both groups (300 diabetics, 5700 normals).

In alcoholics, below the age of 40, the LDL-cholesterol/HDL-cholesterol ratio is very low. There is no overlap with normal blood donors. We can safely say that a ratio below 1.2 rules out a teatotaller. These changes are quickly reversible after cessation of alcohol intake, thus lipoprotein diagnostics can be used for therapeutic monitoring.

Gestagens, for instance Danazol used for treatment of endometriosis, have a strong impact on the lipoprotein profile in an unfavorable direction. HDL are decreased, LDL are increased.

Liver disease is a major cause of all kinds of abnormal lipoproteins. In lipoprotein electrophoresis it often causes a boring pattern: no alpha-lipoproteins and a very broad beta-band. The latter is due to a host of abnormal or abnormally composed lipoproteins. In summary, we find decreased alpha-lipoproteins, a dissociation of A-I and A-II (a rare instance of the presence of LP-A-II) decreased LP-B, abnormal VLDL, poor in Apo-C, remnants in the LDL-class, and LP-X.

Biliary lipids studied in the electron microscope show a bilayered structure. The fingerprint-like structures change drastically if the lipids get into an aqueous environement, such as blood. Stacked discs develop. LP-X has the same appearance. It has the same lipid composition as bile, i. e. no cholesteryl esters, almost no triglycerides, predominantly free cholesterol and phospholipids. In agarose gel it migrates as a beta lipoprotein, thus it is part of the broad beta-band. In agar gel with a high electroendosmosis it migrates towards the cathode and can by this be identified.

LP-X represents most probably a vesicle containing a tiny droplet of plasma. Therefore, one could expect every serum protein to be part of LP-X. What we easily can identify in the polyacrylamide gel electrophoresis are the C-apoproteins, C-I, C-II, and C-III, and the fuzzy band of Apo-D. The albumin band stems from the serum and often is mistaken for Apo-E. Apparently LP-X serves as a nascent lipoprotein and the transferable apoproteins are acquired by or shifted to it and then stick with the particle. Apo-E is a curious exception.

Thus, whenever bile meets blood, LP-X is formed and can be detected by agar electrophoresis.

The VLDL of patients suffering from cholestasis often exhibit beta mobility on agarose gel electrophoresis. This is the second class of lipoproteins present in the broad beta-band. As shown by polyacrylamide gel electrophoresis (3.5%) only the charge but not the size of cholestatic VLDL has changed.

The LDL density class of cholestatic patients often shows a very heterogeneous picture in the electron microscope: normal LP-B particles, the stacked discs of LP-X, and larger spherical particles. These are remnants of triglyceride-rich lipoproteins. LP-B and remnants can be separated from LP-X by Cohn-fractionation and the isolation of remnants can be achieved by immunoaffinity chromatography on an anti-Apo-C column. The remnant contains Apo-B and Apo-C, as demonstrated by immunoelectrophoresis. These particles most probably originate from chylomicrons, since their concentration can be diminished by a fat-free diet.

The presence of the remnants is accompanied by a decrease of the protamine-insensitive postheparin-lipolytic activity. Whether a decrease of the hepatic trigly-ceride lipase is responsible for the diminished remnant catabolism is not clear. It can as well be the decreased rate of hepatic uptake. I will come to this later.

The striking fact of an almost complete absence of alpha-lipoproteins is not accom-panied by a complete lack of the corresponding apolipoproteins. They are decreased, however, and are part of different particles as judged by immunoelectrophoresis against anti-A-I and anti-A-II. After surgical removal of a gallstone, A-I and A-II become part of the same particle.

During the course of recovery from cholestasis major changes are observed in the activity of alkaline phosphatase and gamma-glutamyltransferase and the concentra-tions of bilirubin. Triglycerides decrease, HDL cholesterol and A-I increase, while total cholesterol and Apo-B remain essentially unchanged.

Patients with liver disease usually exhibit low concentrations of apolipoprotein-B. The reason for that is unclear. Decreased food intake may lead to an impaired supply of the liver with cholesterol and subsequent up-regulation of B:E receptors. This may also occur due to impaired fat absorption.

If we consider the several steps of lipoprotein metabolism in which the liver may play a role, we come to the production of lipoproteins, enzymes, and transfer proteins, elimination of unfavorable conditions for lipoprotein metabolism, and receptor-mediated uptake of lipoproteins in the liver.

Impaired hepatic synthesis could be a cause for the low HDL levels. In severe cholestasis fat absorption usually is strongly impaired. This diminishes the contribu-tion of the intestinal synthesis of A-I.

C-II, the activator of lipoprotein lipase, may be sequestered on LP-X. Thus, production of HDL by lipolytic processes may be severely hampered. Lack of C-III, also due to loss to LP-X, may lead to a rapid catabolism of triglyceride-rich lipopro-teins and thus cause a deprivation of the substrate for HDL formation. Lack of C-III may also increase catabolism of HDL particles. Absence of acceptors for Apo-E (TG-rich lipoproteins) from HDL may increase catabolism of HDL particles via B:E- or remnant receptors. Impaired hepatic lipase may lead to abnormal particles with a short life-span. This may be also due to a disturbed exchange of cholesteryl esters and triglycerides.

LP-X is capable of inhibiting the uptake of remnants by the liver of the rat. It therefore may well be responsible for the accumulation of remnants in cholestatic liver disease.

The metabolic consequences of LP-X may be as follows:

1. Abnormal VLDL because of sequestration of Apo-Cs
2. This leads to the formation of lipoproteins which can not well serve as precursors for HDL particles
3. Increased catabolism of several lipoprotein species due to the lack of C-III mediated protection from hepatic uptake by the asialoprotein receptor
4. Induction of hepatic B:E receptors by depleting liver cells of cholesterol
5. Inhibition of the remnant receptor and accumulation of chylomicron remnants in LDL and LP-E in HDL

The clinical usefulness of the LP-X test is well established in the literature. The cumulative specificity is almost 100%. This means that persons without cholestasis can be classified very accurately. Consequently the positive predictive value is almost 100%. This means, the presence of LP-X invariably indicates cholestasis, i.e., the presence of biliary lipids in the blood. The quantitative determination of LP-X is useful in the differentiation of mechanical cholestasis and cholestatic hepatitis. In hepatitis the relative contribution of LP-X to total cholesterol is much higher than in mechanical cholestasis. A high percentage of cholesterol carried by LP-X in combination with a GPT activity below 100 U/l is helpful in ruling out metastatic liver disease.

Turnover Studies of Apolipoproteins C:
A First Critical Appraisal

C. L. Malmendier, and J.-F. Lontie

Introduction

Apolipoproteins of the C group are peptides of small molecular weights, present in chylomicrons, VLDL, IDL, and HDL. These polypeptides have common characteristics: they are regulators (activators or inhibitors) of the lipid metabolism of lipoproteins, particularly the catabolism of triglyceride-rich lipoproteins [1]. The distribution of the different Apo C in lipoprotein classes varies between normal subjects and hypertriglyceridemics and in relation to fasting and the type of diet.

Apo C-I, C-II, and C-III plasma concentrations were determined using different methods (Lowry after IEF, EIA, RIA, or ELISA). Variations between authors may be important for Apo C-II varying between 1 and 3 even in normal subjects [2–18]. The distribution of Apo C between the different lipoproteins can only be compared in healthy fasting subjects. It remains surprising that in these fasting conditions the highest percentage has often been found in VLDL. Evidently, after a 12-h fast, 80% of Apo C are associated with HDL, these particles being predominant in fasting plasma. Already in 1978 Kashyap [19] showed that almost 80% of Apo C-II were associated to HDL in fasting conditions.

Kinetic Experiments of Apo C In Vivo: Experimental Facts

Only a few kinetic studies on Apo C have been realized in vivo in humans [17, 18, 20–23]. Recently, intravenous injection of iodine-labeled Apo C-I, C-II, and C-III, free or associated to HDL, has allowed to quantification of the metabolism of each apoprotein in healthy volunteers.

First, free iodine-labeled Apo C-II and Apo C-III were injected intravenously into normal human subjects. The very high specific activity of the tracer made it possible to follow the different lipoprotein decay curves for as long as 15 days which is in contrast to other studies lasting only 2 or 4 days. As all activity injected was confined to a single apoprotein, no further isolation procedure was required, which very much increased the accuracy of the specific apoprotein measurement.

The plasma decay curves of Apo C-I, C-II, and C-III shown on Fig. 1 seem comparable in normal subjects. The decay of the three Apo Cs is faster than that of Apo A-I, but even between the Cs, C-III decrease is quicker than Apo C-I and Apo C-II decrease. Radioactivity was determined directly in total plasma and in the VLDL, IDL+LDL, HDL and d 1.25 infranate without further processing of the

H. U. Klör (Ed.)
Lipoprotein Subfractions
Omega-3 Fatty Acids
© Springer-Verlag Berlin Heidelberg 1989

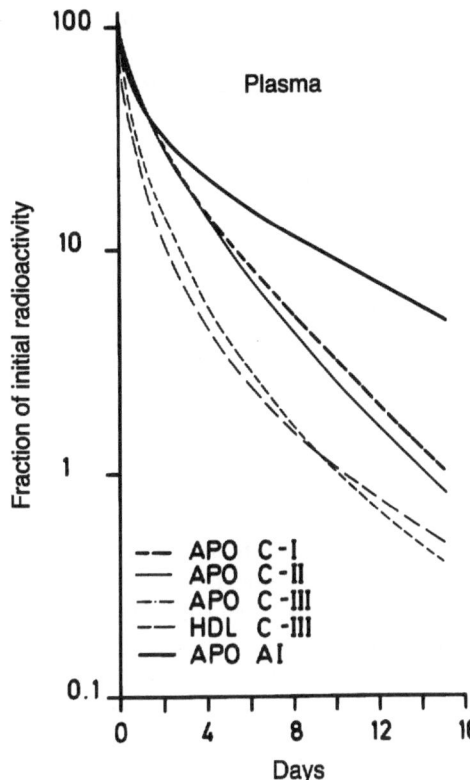

Fig. 1. Plasma radioactivity decay curves of apolipoproteins C-I, C-II, and C-III (compared with apo A-I) as a function of time

samples. We observed that the decay curves of all lipoprotein fractions were parallel from the first day.

Mathematical analysis of the plasma curves (total radioactivity) was made using a three-compartmental model (known as Matthews's model). This analysis allowed calculation of the "global" kinetic parameters describing Apo C metabolism. FCR (fractional catabolic rate) (0.422 ± 0.044 and 0.455 ± 0.091 pool/day) and mean residence times through the system (3.24 ± 0.27 and 3.30 ± 1.00 days) for Apo C-I and Apo C-II, respectively, are very close, and the difference in production rates (1.79 ± 0.18 and 0.63 ± 0.17 mg/kg · day) results from their respective plasma concentrations (10.3 ± 0.6 and 3.4 ± 1.3 mg/dl). The FCR of Apo C-III (0.767 ± 0.125) is much higher and residence times thus shorter (2.45 ± 0.33 days); the synthesis rate is 2.28 ± 0.32 mg/kg · day. Different parameters mean different metabolism between Apo C-I and C-II, on one hand, and Apo C-III, on the other.

Kinetics and Modelling

The notion of kinetics of a lipoprotein particle as a whole becomes vague when all of its components can undergo transitions independently, unless it contains at least one marker with which it can be totally identified [24]

For Apo C, two conflicting tendencies have become manifest, both based on experimental data. Some authors have found specific activities to be identical (or very close) for the different lipoprotein families, whereas others have observed important differences in specific activities. These two observations have resulted from in vivo experiments involving almost exclusively intravenous injections of VLDL in vitro labeled with iodine (exogenous labeling). Huff et al. [20, 21] found comparable Apo C-II and C-III specific activities in both VLDL and HDL, though very slightly higher in VLDL. Bukberg et al. [25] found that after injection of 125-iodine labeled VLDL, Apo C-III specific activities were slightly higher in VLDL than in HDL (these results are similar to those of Huff and Nestel), but, surprisingly, after injecting labeled HDL during a 96 h experiment, they observed specific activities two times higher in HDL than in VLDL and came to the conclusion that nonexchangeable pools exist in both VLDL and HDL.

Those who observed identical or close specific activities have not seen the necessity to build a complex compartmental model, and have adopted a two- or three-compartmental model [20, 21, 25], applicable to a homogeneous particle.

At the other end of the spectrum, Berman described different kinetics for ApoC-VLDL and ApoC-HDL as accounting for different specific activities. He constructed a compartmental model of lipoprotein kinetics from data observed for Apo B kinetic behavior [22]. This model displays the importance of a stepwise delipidation chain in VLDL. The Apo B is considered to be a structural component carrying lipid (essentially triglycerides at the VLDL stage) and associated temporarily to other apoproteins (C and E). Based on this Apo B model, he proposed an analogous model for Apo C [22], adding a subsystem for HDL-C but deleting the LDL subsystem. Observations showed that the Apo C remain associated to VLDL for a limited time, i. e., during the triglyceride hydrolysis described in the model by the delipidation cascade leading to the conversion of VLDL to IDL and finally to LDL.

Berman's model nevertheless poses major problems:

1. The necessity to add an x-VLDL radioactivity attributed in part to lipid label or to partially denatured material (x is external to the main exchange processes)
2. The delay observed in the x-VLDL-C recycling pathway
3. The presence of an important initial labeling in HDL-C in the first sample (10 min) after injection of labeled VLDL alone
4. The impossibility to determine the entry site (HDL or VLDL) of newly synthesized Apo C
5. The absence of direct determination of Apo C concentrations in total plasma and lipoprotein fractions
6. The absence of values for individual Apo C components

This model leads to different specific activities in the different compartments. However, it is not possible to neglect the very quick exchanges between lipoproteins, which was not taken into account by Berman and his team. We tried to fit to the same model the data obtained after injection of labeled free apolipoprotein C-III [23]. A good fit was obtained for the radioactivity curves of HDL, VLDL, and IDL using parameter values in the same range as Berman, but with the necessary addition of three compartments, one for each type of lipoprotein, called x, and applicable to the initial activity observed in HDL in Berman's experiments. These x values were so preponderant that the model becomes meaningless. Our HDL-Apo C three-compartmental subsystem was able to absorb all perturbations of the steady-state amounts of Apo C in the different pools. Owing to the absence of physiological significance of the x compartments and to the inconsistencies appearing during the tentative fitting of the steady-states (negative values of the fluxes for some exchanges), we had to look for another explanation. The difficulties encountered in fitting obviously resulted also from the fact that the rates of exchange were much faster than was anticipated from the model and incited us to restate the problem of specific activities. In addition, all these calculations are based on identical kinetics for Apo C-II and C-III.

In Vitro Experiments

In order to gain some information about the order of magnitude of the in vitro exchange rates between lipoproteins, two assays were performed on a Superose 6 FPLC chromatography column (total elution time, 3 h).

First, labeled HDL-Apo C-III were put down onto the surface of the gel, and less than 1 min later, unlabeled VLDL+IDL (d < 1.019 g/ml) was injected. With VLDL eluting in the void volume and HDL moving much more slowly, through the gel, their contact was actually very limited in time. A significant amount of activity associated to VLDL (31.6%) and IDL (52.3%), while only 14.9% remained with HDL.

Second, labeled HDL-Apo C-III were mixed with 1 ml plasma, and immediately put down onto the surface of the gel. The distribution of activity between lipoproteins was similar to that observed after a much longer incubation.

These results imply that a very quick exchange (less than 1 min) takes place in vitro between lipoproteins related to the relative proportion of native lipoproteins. Exchange, however, does not necessarily mean true equilibrium between the fractions. In vitro experiments of incubation of labeled Apo C with plasma showed that the exchange of radioactivity between the lipoprotein fractions seemed fast and independent of the incubation time. Actually no difference in distribution appeared for incubation times varying from 10 min to 4 h. The exchanges between lipoproteins may not be really blocked in the experimental test tube after sampling. Moreover, equilibration has plenty of time to take place during storage and processing of the sample. In this closed system, thus, the equilibrium of the tracer (free labeled Apo C) seemed immediate.

In the in vivo experiments as well (open system) the radioactivity appears to equilibrate quickly (from the 10-min sample after injection) between the different classes of lipoproteins in a ratio similar to that observed in vitro. These observations concerned all kinetic experiments on Apo C performed using labeled lipoproteins (VLDL or HDL), experiments requiring separation of plasma, isolation of lipoproteins by long-lasting ultracentrifugation and/or chromatography. It is therefore impossible to have experimentally access to the real percentage of partition present immediately at the moment of the sampling in fixing the situation either in vitro or in vivo.

In in vitro incubation experiments with Apo C (VLDL or HDL) in the presence of pathological plasma, the ratio between the amounts of labeled lipoproteins and

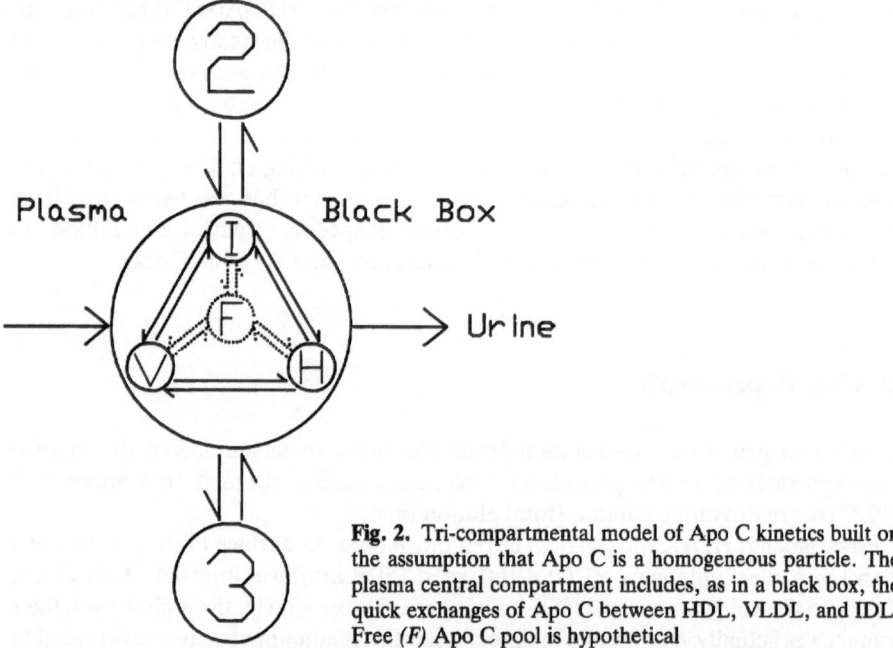

Fig. 2. Tri-compartmental model of Apo C kinetics built on the assumption that Apo C is a homogeneous particle. The plasma central compartment includes, as in a black box, the quick exchanges of Apo C between HDL, VLDL, and IDL. Free *(F)* Apo C pool is hypothetical

plasma lipoproteins becomes crucial, due to the qualitative changes (lipid/lipid and lipid/protein ratios) and the quantitative changes in the lipoproteins of these abnormal plasma. After a 30-min incubation, the equilibrium between specific activities is not completely reached.

After having demonstrated that a very quick equilibrium of Apo C specific activities takes place in vitro and essentially in vivo in normal plasma, we were obliged to come back to a simple tri-compartmental model (Fig. 2). The central plasma compartment is a black box in which very quick exchanges, compared to the frequency of sampling, take place between VLDL, IDL, and HDL. A schematic representation analogous to the one we have developed has been published in 1978 by Schaefer et al. [1]. There is no evidence for the existence of a "free" pool of Apo C.

Discussion

Effect of Ultracentrifugation

In our in vivo experiments on normal subjects, the specific activity is identical for HDL and VLDL. One may question whether this represents a physiological fact or an artifact related to the methods used for the measurements. It is known that ultracentrifugation per se alters the apoprotein composition of lipoproteins, loosening in particular some Apo C from VLDL and from HDL. Nevertheless, if it is true that in our studies the ultracentrifugation caused an increase of the Apo C radioactivity in the bottom (d > 1.25 g/ml), the distribution between lipoprotein fractions appeared not much affected when we compared the distribution obtained after chromatography before and after a single ultracentrifugation step [18]. Thus, ultracentrifugation undoubtedly unbinds some Apo C from both VLDL and HDL but does not modify significantly the distribution of radioactivity between lipoprotein fractions.

Influence of the Method Used for the Determination of the Apo C Mass

Differences in specific activities may result from the method of determination of the tracee. Apoprotein concentrations used by Berman et al. in the building of their model were indirect, deriving from measured cholesterol and triglyceride values and from measured or published composition data on each class of particles [22]. No attempt was made to measure individually Apo C-II and Apo C-III. Huff and Nestel [20, 21] also used an indirect method consisting of isoelectric focusing of apoproteins followed by densitometric scanning and slicing of polyacrylamide gels. Bukberg et al. [11] determined Apo C-III by a more specific method (Lowry and RIA) after separation by affinity chromatography (anti-Apo C-III Sepharose column) of Apo C-III peptides coming from delipidated lipoprotein fractions.

At least the first two procedures may lead to considerable errors. We are of the opinion that the metabolic pool masses were not at all accurately estimated. In order to reduce this methodological error to a minimum, we used specific sandwich ELISA directly on the lipoprotein fractions.

Dynamics of Apo C Exchanges

Two apolipoprotein exchange processes between lipoproteins must be considered:
1. Quick and spontaneous "passive" exchanges without apoprotein mass transfer, with the amount of Apo C leaving one particle to automatically replaced by an equivalent amount coming from another lipoprotein particle. This reflects the system equilibrium as long as it is not perturbed by both alimentary intestinal input and hepatic release of triglyceride-rich lipoproteins. These exchange rates may not be experimentally determined with precision in vivo. The exchanges maintain a dynamic association-dissociation equilibrium between the different lipoproteins as a function of their relative concentrations in plasma. The specific configuration of lipids at the surface of lipoprotein determines the association constant. It is possible that Apo C may be accompanied by phospholipids during this exchange. A spontaneous transfer of phospholipids may potentially exist but would be too slow, according to Massey et al. [26] to be a physiologically important phenomenon. This transfer probably occurs by diffusion of monomeric phospholipid molecules through the aqueous phase, owing to desorption proportional to the degree of hydrophobicity of phospholipid fatty acid chain [27]. Plasma PTP (phospholipid transfer protein) [27] or LTP-2 (lipid transfer protein) [28] facilitate the transfer of phospholipids between HDL and VLDL. Until now, it has not been determined that Apo C participates in this phospholipid transfer.
2. "Active exchange" or net mass transfer. (a) The entry into circulation of native VLDL (or chylomicrons) produces an Apo C transfer from the HDL to VLDL

pool. The affinity of VLDL-TG for Apo C is high. The mechanism of this transfer is not well understood. Thermodynamically it is impossible for Apo C to exist in free form in plasma [29]; Apo C would be linked to lipids, most likely to phospholipids. (b) As lipolysis goes on, there is an "active" return of Apo C from VLDL and IDL to HDL. VLDL will give birth to two types of particles, particles similar to HDL, containing PL, TG, and Apo C, which will mix with the HDL pool [30], and particles containing Apo B100, a small amount of Apo C, TG, and PL, that as they convert to IDL will lose their load in Apo C before being taken up by hepatic and peripheral Apo B, E receptors. A similar mechanism will operate for chylomicrons. Lipolysis of chylomicrons will give remnants rich in Apo E, Apo B-48, and TG which will be cleared at the level of receptors, but also particles rich in Apo A-I, Apo A-II, C and in PL that will combine with the HDL pool [31].

A schematic representation of these metabolic events is shown in Fig. 3.

Metabolic Specificity of Apo C

Although the metabolic role of Apo C-I is still unknown, the fact that a correlation exists between its plasma VLDL distribution and hypertriglyceridemia [6] suggests that Apo C-I will leave VLDL spontaneously during the delipidation cascade to HDL.

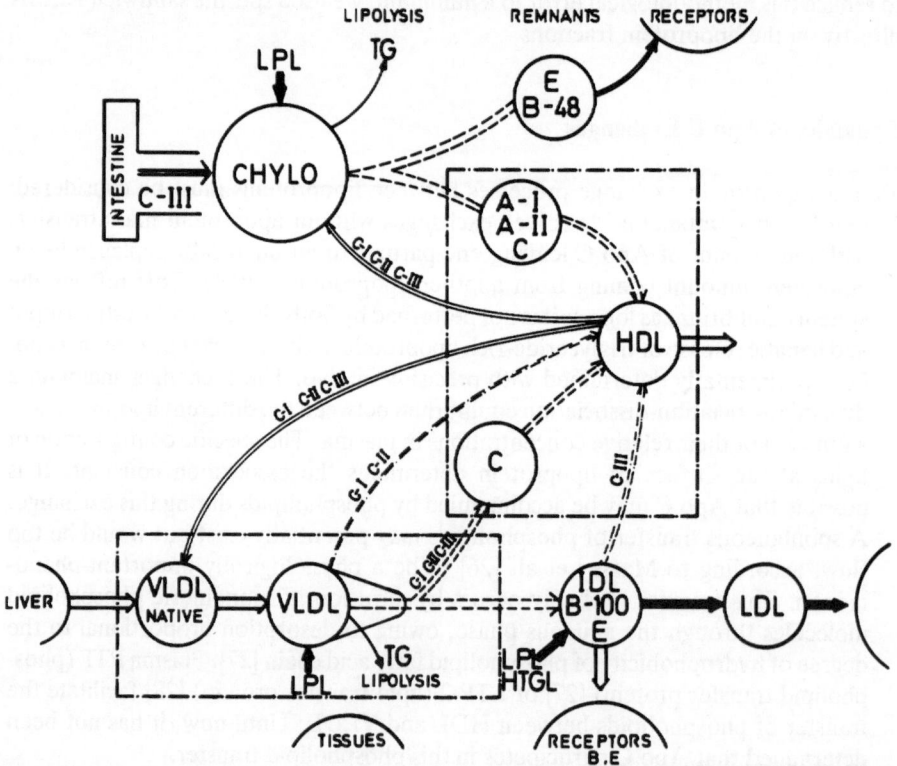

Fig. 3. Schematic representation of Apo C metabolic events. *LPL*, lipoprotein lipase; *HTGL*, hepatic triglyceride lipase

In a similar way, Apo C-II and Apo C-III are transferred from VLDL to HDL during lipolysis. Apo C-II is linked to lipoprotein lipase by a protein-protein interaction at the site of hydrolysis after penetration of LPL into the phospholipid monolayer [32], a lipid binding to Apo C-II not being needed for the activating effect. Apo C-III will act as a competitive inhibitor at the stage of linkage of Apo C with LPL. As VLDL is impoverished in triglyceride by triglyceridasic action and in PL by phospholipasic action [33], Apo C-II leaves the particle and returns to HDL. Apo C-III may remain longer on the particle with phospholipids and inhibit the uptake of remnants, as long as part of the phosphatidylcholine has not been hydrolyzed to lysophosphatidyl-choline (LPC) [34]. LPC will favor the departure of Apo C-III and the remnant will be able to bind to the Apo B, E receptor [34].

Triglyceride hydrolysis at the different steps of the delipidation cascade does not strictly parallel phospholipid hydrolysis. Since the affinity of the different Apo C for lipoproteins is a function of the lipid environment, it is likely that transfers of C-II and C-III also are not parallel.

The metabolic differences between the different Apo C may be due to:

1. A difference at the level of synthesis. Coding genes for C-I and C-II [35] are close on chromosome 19, whereas coding genes of Apo C-III and Apo A-I are close on chromosome 11 [36]. It is likely that independently of Apo C-III, Apo C-I and C-II biosynthesis is coordinately controled. Deficiencies of both Apo C-I and C-II [37], and deficiencies of Apo A-I and C-III [38] have been described and attributed to a common anomaly of their biosynthesis regulatory process at the gene level.

2. A difference at the catabolic level. The plasma decay curves of Apo C-I and C-II are comparable, whereas Apo C-III decays faster. Evidence of the catabolic difference is the shape of the urinary/plasma (U/P) ratio curve, which suggests a metabolic heterogeneity at least for lipoprotein particles containing Apo C-III (Fig. 4). The U/P ratio remains rather stable from day 8 to day 16 after tracer injection (Fig. 4).

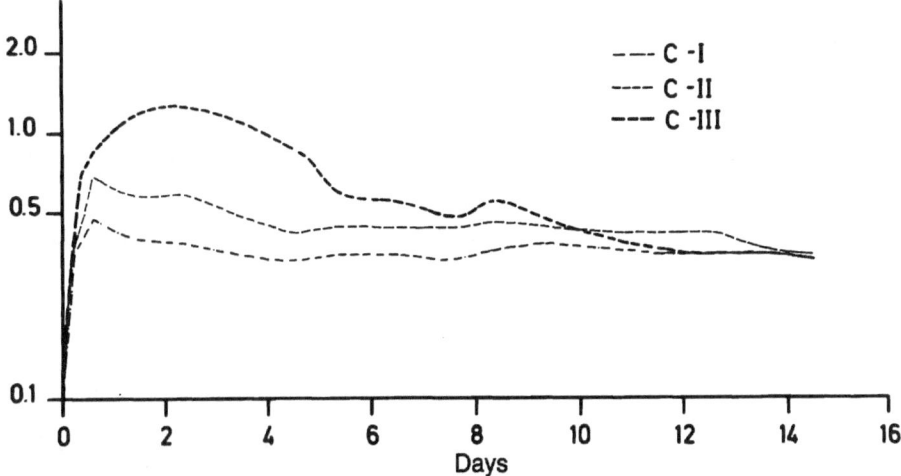

Fig. 4. Urine/plasma *(U/P)* activity ratio as a function of time

Alaupovic, in a paper with Puchois and Fruchart [39], proposed the existence of particles containing A-I:C-I:C-II and others containing A-I:B:C-III and A-I:E:C-III in the HDL class. Earlier, Alaupovic [40] had also demonstrated the existence of B:E:C-I:C-II:C-III and B:E:C-III particles. In addition, the variation in C-II/C-III ratio in hypertriglyceridemics [41, 42] and in renal insufficiency ([43] and [44] C.L. Malmendier, J.F. Lontie, unpublished observations) suggest differences in metabolism for Apo C-II and C-III.

Conclusions

1. Kinetic studies were made of Apo C in normal subjects. It was impossible to build a complex compartmental model quantifying the exchanges between lipoproteins, since quick passive exchanges were not experimentally separable from exchanges involving mass transfer appearing with the entry of chylomicron or native VLDL into circulation. The kinetics of individual lipoproteins for Apo C were thus illusory.
2. Global kinetics, however, allowed calculation of some parameters in normal volunteers, i.e., fractional catabolic rate, rate of synthesis, and mean residence time determined by the mathematical analysis of both plasma decay curves and urinary excretion rates. Such studies demonstrated different metabolisms for Apo C-I, C-II, and C-III. They may supply essential information on the perturbations observed in pathology.
3. Since lipid transfer proteins were demonstrated, it will be essential to demonstrate the common route of Apo C and phospholipids (with a specificity for each Apo C), when VLDL undergo lipolysis. The mechanism of Apo C transfer from HDL to triglyceride-rich lipoproteins (VLDL or chylomicrons) remains obscure.
4. The data coming from in vitro incubation studies must be interpreted with caution before being extrapolated to in vivo physiological mechanisms, as they involve a closed system, with limited enzymatic activities, with the absence of turnover – in the presence of a limited size of distribution volume for the tracer.

References

1. Schaefer EJ, Eisenberg S, Levy RI (1978) Lipoprotein apoprotein metabolism. J Lipid Res 19: 667–687
2. Kashyap ML, Srivastava LS, Chen CY, Perisutti G, Campbell M, Lutmer RF, Glueck CJ (1977) Radioimmunoassay of human apolipoprotein C-II. A study in normal and hypertriglyceridemic subjects. J Clin Invest 60: 171–180
3. Schonfeld G, George PK, Miller J, Reilly P, Witztum J (1979) Apolipoprotein C-II and C-III levels in hyperlipoproteinemia. Metabolism 28: 1001–1010
4. Kashyap ML, Srivastava LS, Hynd BA, Gartside PS, Perisutti G (1981) Quantitation of human apolipoprotein C-III and its subspecies by radioimmunoassay and analytical isoelectric focusing: abnormal plasma triglyceride-rich lipoprotein apolipoprotein C-III subspecies concentrations in hypertriglyceridemia. J Lipid Res 22: 800–810
5. Barr SI, Kottke BA, Mao SJT (1985) Postprandial distribution of apolipoproteins C-II and C-III in normal subjects and patients with mild hypertriglyceridemia: comparison of meals containing corn oil and medium-chain triglyceride oil. Metabolism 34: 983–992

6. Polz E, Kotite L, Havel RJ, Kane JP, Sata T (1980) Human apolipoprotein C-I: concentration in blood serum and lipoproteins. Biochem Med 24: 229–237
7. Curry MD, McConathy WJ, Fesmire JD, Alaupovic P (1980) Quantitative determination of human apolipoprotein C-III by electroimmunoassay. Biochim Biophys Acta 617: 503–513
8. Barr SI, Kottke BA, Chang JY, Mao SJT (1981) Immunochemistry of human plasma apolipoprotein C-II as studied by radioimmunoassay. Biochim Biophys Acta 663: 491–505
9. Curry MD, McConathy WJ, Fesmire JD, Alaupovic P (1981) Quantitative determination of apolipoproteins C-I and C-II in human plasma by separate electroimmunoassays. Clin Chem 27: 543–548
10. Carlson LA, Holmquist L (1982) Concentrations of apolipoproteins B, C-I, C-II, C-III and E in sera from normal men and their relation to serum lipoprotein levels. Clin Chim Acta 124: 163–178
11. Bukberg PR, Le N-A, Ginsberg HN, Gibson JC, Goldman LC, Brown WV (1983) Direct measurement of apolipoprotein C-III specific activity in ^{125}I-labeled very low density lipoproteins using immunoaffinity chromatography. J Lipid Res 24: 1251–1260
12. Gustafson S, Ostlund-Lindqvist, Vessby B (1984) A rapid radioimmunoassay of human apolipoproteins C-II and C-III. Scand J Clin Lab Invest 44: 291–297
13. Weisweiler P, Schwandt P (1984) Determination of human apolipoproteins C-II and C-III by laser nephelometry. Fresenius Z Anal Chem 317: 708–709
14. Bury J, Rosseneu M (1985) Enzyme linked immunosorbent assay for human apolipoprotein C-III. J Clin Chem Clin Biochem 23: 63–68
15. Bury J, Michiels G, Rosseneu M (1986) Human apolipoprotein C-II quantitation by sandwich enzyme-linked immunosorbent assay. J Clin Chem Clin Biochem 24: 457–463
16. Riesen WF, Sturzenegger E (1986) Enzyme-linked immunosorbent assay for apolipoprotein C-I. J Clin Chem Clin Biochem 24: 723–727
17. Malmendier CL, Lontie J-F, Grutman GA, Delcroix C (1986) Metabolism of apolipoprotein C-I in normolipoproteinemic human subjects. Atherosclerosis 62: 167–172
18. Malmendier CL, Lontie J-F, Grutman GA, Delcroix C (1988) Metabolism of apolipoprotein C-III in normolipemic human subjects. Atherosclerosis 69: 51–59
19. Kashyap ML, Srivastava LS, Hynd BA, Perisutti G, Brady DW, Gartside P, Glueck CJ (1978) The role of high density lipoprotein apolipoprotein C-II in triglyceride metabolism. Lipids 13: 933–942
20. Huff MW, Nestel PJ (1982) Metabolism of apolipoproteins C-II, C-III$_1$, C-III$_2$ and VLDL-B in human subjects consuming high carbohydrate diets. Metabolism 31: 493–498
21. Huff MW, Fidge NH, Nestel PJ, Billington T, Watson B (1981) Metabolism of C-apolipoproteins: kinetics of C-II, C-III$_1$ and C-III$_2$, and VLDL-apolipoprotein B in normal and hyperlipoproteinemic subjects. J Lipid Res 22: 1235–1246
22. Berman M, Hall M III, Levy RI, Eisenberg S, Bilheimer DW, Phair RD, Goebel RH (1978) Metabolism of ApoB and ApoC lipoproteins in man: kinetic studies in normal and hyperlipoproteinemic subjects. J Lipid Res 19: 38–56
23. Malmendier CL, Lontie J-F, Grutman G, Delcroix C (1987) Metabolism of apolipoprotein C: kinetic studies in human subjects: a critical review. In: Malmendier CL, Alaupovic P (eds) Lipoproteins and atherosclerosis. Plenum, New York, pp 95–103
24. Berman M (1982) Kinetic analysis and modeling: theory and applications to lipoproteins. In: Berman M, Grundy SM, Howard BV (eds) Lipoprotein kinetics and modeling. Academic, New York, pp 3–36
25. Bukberg PR, Le N-A, Ginsberg HN, Gibson JC, Rubinstein A, Brown WV (1985) Evidence for non-equilibrating pools of apolipoprotein C-III in plasma lipoproteins. J Lipid Res 26: 1047–1057
26. Massey JB, Hickson D, She HS, Sparrow JT, Via DP, Gotto AM Jr, Pownall HJ (1984) Measurement and prediction rates of spontaneous transfer of phospholipids between plasma lipoproteins. Biochim Biophys Acta 794: 274–280
27. Tall AR (1986) Plasma lipid transfer proteins. J Lipid Res 27: 361–367
28. Albers JJ, Tollefson JH, Chen C-H, Steinmetz A (1984) Isolation and characterization of human plasma lipid transfer proteins. Arteriosclerosis 4: 49–58
29. Dolphin PJ (1985) Lipoprotein metabolism and the role of apolipoproteins as metabolic programmers. Can J Biochem Cell Biol 63: 850–869

30. Tam SP, Breckenridge WC (1983) Apolipoprotein and lipid distribution between vesicles and HDL-like particles formed during lipolysis of human very low density lipoproteins by perfused rat heart. J Lipid Res 24: 1343–1357
31. Schaefer EJ, Wetzel MG, Bengtsson G, Scow RO, Brewer HB Jr, Olivecrona T (1982) Transfer of human lymph chylomicron constituents to other lipoprotein density fractions during in vitro lipolysis. J Lipid Res 23: 1259–1273
32. Vainio P, Virtanen JA, Kinnunen PKJ, Voyta JC, Smith LC, Gotto AM Jr, Sparrow JT, Pattus F, Verger R (1983) Action of lipoprotein lipase on phospholipid monolayers. Activation by apolipoprotein C-II. Biochemistry 22: 2270–2275
33. Shirai K, Fitzharris TJ, Shinomiya M, Muntz HG, Harmony JAK, Jackson RL, Quinn DM (1983) Lipoprotein lipase-catalysed hydrolysis of phosphatidylcholine of guinea pig very low density lipoproteins and discoidal complexes of phospholipid and apolipoprotein: effect of apolipoprotein C-II on the catalytic mechanism. J Lipid Res 24: 721–730
34. Windler EET, Preyer S, Greten H (1986) Influence of lysophosphatidyl-choline on the C-apolipoprotein content of rat and human triglyceride-rich lipoproteins during triglyceride hydrolysis. J Clin Invest 78: 658–665
35. Scott J, Knott TJ, Shaw DJ, Brook JD (1985) Localization of genes encoding apolipoproteins C-I, C-II, and E to the p13-cen region of human chromosome 19. Hum Genet 71: 144–146
36. Law SW, Gray G, Brewer HB Jr, Sakaguchi AY, Naylor SL (1984) Human apolipoprotein A-I and C-III genes reside in the p11–q13 region of chromosome 11. Biochem Biophys Res Commun 118: 934–942
37. Dumon M-F, Clerc M (1986) Preliminary report on a case of apolipoproteins C-I and C-II deficiency. Clin Chim Acta 157: 239–248
38. Norum RA, Lakier JB, Goldstein S, Angel A, Goldberg RB, Block WD, Noffze DK, Dolphin PJ, Edelglass J, Bogorad DD, Alaupovic P (1982) Familial deficiency of apolipoproteins A-I and C-III and precocious coronary-artery disease. N Engl J Med 306: 1513–1519
39. Puchois P, Alaupovic P, Fruchart JC (1985) Mise au point sur les classifications des lipoprotéines plasmatiques. Ann Biol Clin (Paris) 43: 831–840
40. Alaupovic P, Tavella M, Fesmire J (1987) Separation and identification of Apo-B-containing lipoprotein particles in normolipidemic subjects and patients with hyperlipoproteinemias. In: Malmendier CL, Alaupovic P (eds) Lipoproteins and atherosclerosis. Plenum, New York, pp 7–14
41. Carlson LA, Ballantyne D (1976) Changing relative proportions of apolipoproteins C-II and C-III of very low density lipoproteins in hypertriglyceridemia. Atherosclerosis 23: 563–568
42. Erkelens DW, Mocking JAJ (1982) The C-II/C-III ratio of transferable apolipoprotein in primary and secondary hypertriglyceridemia. Clin Chim Acta 121: 56–65
43. Attman PO, Gustafson A, Alaupovic P, Knight C, Wang CS, Bass H (1980) Abnormalities of plasma, lipoprotein system in patients with chronic renal failure. Circulation 62: 118

Lecithin: Cholesterol Acyl Transferase, Cholesterol Ester Exchange/Transfer Protein, and Lipoprotein Particles

G. M. Kostner, and E. Steyrer

Introduction

More than 80% of the cholesteryl esters (CE) found in human plasma derive from the reaction of lecithin: cholesterol acyl transferase (LCAT). Since the content of CE in plasma high positively correlates with the incidence of atherosclerosis and myocardial infarction, there has been in the past and still is great interest in investigation of the enzymes involved in lipoprotein metabolism. This overview summarizes some general features, with particular emphasis on investigations carried out in our laboratory: (a) the substrates of LCAT in plasma; (b) the influence of LCAT on the lipoprotein spectrum; (c) the distribution of formed CE after the action of LCAT; (d) the impact of cholesteryl ester transfer/exchange protein (CETP) on lipoprotein metabolism.

Substrates of LCAT in Plasma

LCAT Reaction and Physiological Substrate of LCAT

LCAT catalyzes the transfer reaction of unsaturated fatty acids in position II of lecithin (PC) to free cholesterol (FC), giving rise to the formation of CE and lysolecithin. LCAT does not act on artificial lipid emulsions containing PC and FC without any apolipoprotein, but there exist some cofactors which catalyze the above reaction [1].

It is believed that in human plasma the so-called nascent HDL, which consists of a disk-like lipoprotein, is the major substrate of LCAT. During the reaction of LCAT, CE, the core lipid, is formed, which converts this disk-shaped lipoprotein into spherical HDL [2].

Role of the Cholesterol Ester Transfer/Exchange Protein

It is generally accepted that CE, which is formed in HDL does not remain there. It is transferred to triglyceride-rich lipoproteins and to CE-rich lipoproteins (VLDL and LDL). This reaction is catalyzed by specific transfer or exchange proteins called cholesteryl ester transfer/exchange proteins (CETP). There are probably several different specific proteins, which catalyze the transfer of these core lipids and of surface lipids from HDL to VLDL and LDL [3].

H. U. Klör (Ed.)
Lipoprotein Subfractions
Omega-3 Fatty Acids
© Springer-Verlag Berlin Heidelberg 1989

LCAT Activators

The major LCAT activator is apolipoprotein A-I (ApoA-I) [4], but it has been postulated also that other apolipoproteins may activate LCAT, e. g., the apoproteins C-I, A-IV, and E. We have previously reported that ApoD also activates LCAT, but studies from another laboratory have challenged our proposal. Therefore, we have reinvestigated this problem [5].

As can be seen in Fig. 1, ApoD in fact activates LCAT. The reactivity of ApoD, expressed as fractional esterification rate (FER) per incubation time, is about 30% that of ApoA-I. The reaction proceeds linearly up to 60 min, whereas in proteoliposomes with ApoA-I, FER increases faster, but then the curve levels off. One possible explanation of this might be that ApoD stabilizes the LCAT during this reaction.

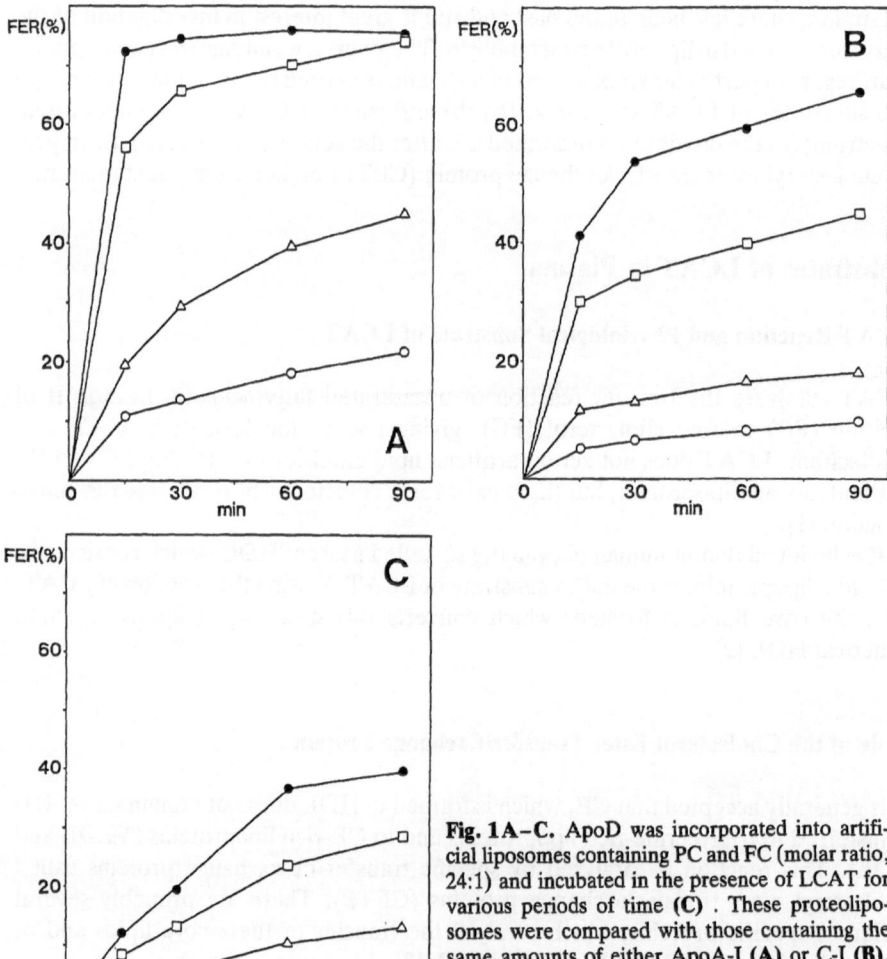

Fig. 1A–C. ApoD was incorporated into artificial liposomes containing PC and FC (molar ratio, 24:1) and incubated in the presence of LCAT for various periods of time **(C)** . These proteoliposomes were compared with those containing the same amounts of either ApoA-I **(A)** or C-I **(B)**. Apoprotein concentrations (in µg/ml) were 10 *(circles)*, 30 *(triangles)*, 100 *(squares)*, or 30 *(filled circles)*

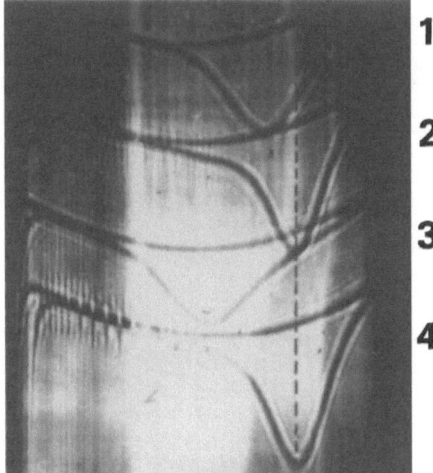

Fig. 2. Schlieren pattern of several HDL fractions isolated after 24-h incubation of plasma. From *top* to *bottom: (1)* Total HDL isolated from normal fasting plasma incubated at 37°C; *(2)* reference plasma stored at 4°C; *(3)* plasma incubated at 37°C in the presence of triglyceride (TG)-rich lipoproteins; *(4)* same as *(3)* but after inhibition of LCAT with 5 mM iodoacetate

Influence of LCAT on the Lipoprotein Spectrum

Incubation of Whole Serum with Active LCAT

In order to get an answer to the question, what happens in vivo, when LCAT is acting, we incubated whole plasma in the presence of active LCAT, or alternatively LCAT was inhibited by the addition of 5 mM iodoacetate [6]. After incubation for 24 h at 37°C, several lipoprotein density fractions were separated by ultrazentrifugation (Fig. 2).

If LCAT acts in fasting plasma, HDL-3 shifts slightly towards the density of HDL-2a. After the addition of TG-rich lipoproteins, e.g., chylomicrons, VLDL, or intralipid, we found a complete conversion of HDL towards HDL-2b. This, however, occurs only if LCAT is active.

Incubation with Isolated HDL Subfractions

Similar experiments were performed with purified HDL and VLDL plus pure LCAT and/or CETP (Fig. 3).

After addition of LCAT plus CETP the whole HDL-3 is converted to HDL-2. This conversion was not seen after incubation of HDL-3 with LCAT or CETP alone.

We concluded from these results that LCAT, CETP, and TG-rich lipoproteins are necessary for the formation of HDL-2.

Influence of LCAT on LDL

Similar experiments as for HDL were also carried out with LDL. The flotation rate of LCAT-treated LDL varies depending on the lipoproteins additionally present in the

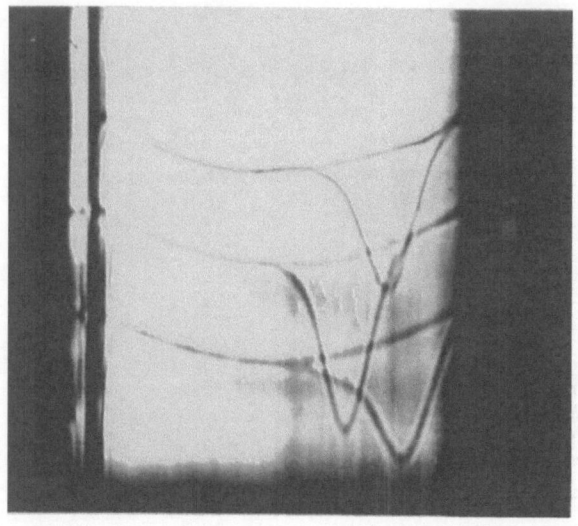

1

2

3

Fig. 3. HDL plusVLDL (ratio 1:5) were incubated with purified LCAT and CETP. From *top* to *bottom:* *(1)* Total HDL fraction isolated after incubation of HDL-3 + VLDL in the presence of CETP; *(2)* same as *(1)* but + active LCAT; *(3)* control total HDL from fasting plasma

incubation mixture. LDL, incubated in the presence of TG-rich lipoproteins or with hypertriglyceridemic plasma, migrates electrophoretically faster than the reference LDL.

Metabolism of LCAT-Treated LDL

The LCAT-treated LDL differs from that of reference LDL in chemical composition as well as the content of non-ApoB proteins. The LCAT-modified LDL isolated from plasma after incubation for 24 h had a much higher content of apoproteins C, E, A-I, and A-II.

LCAT treatment of LDL reduced its binding and internalization into cultured human fibroblasts, whereas the degradation was increased [7] (Fig. 4).

Influence of LCAT on LDL Metabolism In Vivo

LCAT-treated LDL was labelled with 125-I and reference-LDL with 131-I; both LDLs were injected intravenously into five volunteers. A slight but significant difference in the catabolic rate was seen: the LCAT-treated LDL was catabolized more slowly than the reference LDL [8].

Experiments wit Pig Plasma

Role of CETP

Pig is an animal species which, in contrast to humans, lacks cholesterol ester transfer/exchange activity (CETA). Thus, study of pig plasma provided an opportunity to

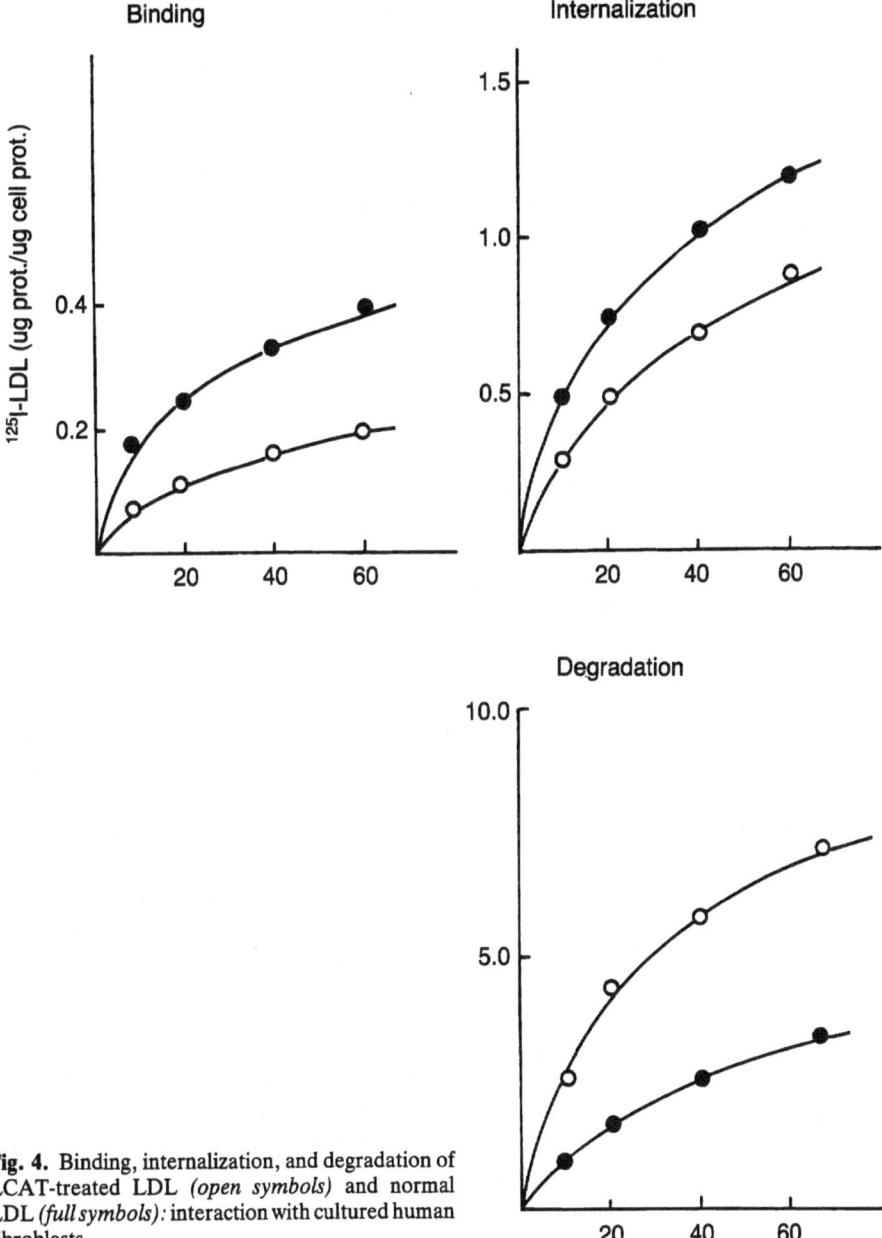

Fig. 4. Binding, internalization, and degradation of LCAT-treated LDL *(open symbols)* and normal LDL *(full symbols):* interaction with cultured human fibroblasts

support our findings in humans, namely that CETP might be responsible for the formation of HDL-2 in concert with TG-rich lipoproteins and LCAT.

While similar incubation experiments as described above were performed with the bottom fraction of pig plasma, a conversion of HDL-3 to HDL-2b was not observed [9].

Origin of CE in Porcine LDL

Since the pig lacks CETA, the question arose concerning the origin of CE found in LDL of this species. We tested the possibility that LDL itself may be a substrate of LCAT.

Pig LDL at different purification stages were incubated with pure LCAT and the esterification of free cholesterol was compared with that of pig HDL. It was found that LDL isolated by ultracentrifugation, which contained traces of ApoA-I and ApoC, yielded cholesterol esterification in the order of 30% that of HDL. If, on the other hand, completely pure LDL was enriched with PC by incubation with PC:FC-liposomes, the newly formed LDL was as good a substrate of LCAT as HDL.

From these results we conclude, that the core lipids in LDL are synthesized by the direct action of LCAT on this lipoprotein fraction [10].

Impact of CETP on Lipoprotein Metabolism

CETA and Plasma HDL Levels

It is believed that nascent HDL are formed in the liver, and during a complex reaction in which TG-rich lipoproteins, lipoprotein lipase, LCAT, and CETP are involved, a given HDL pattern is created with a fixed HDL2/3 ratio. To what extent CETP activity may influence the HDL concentration, or vice versa, was unknown.

We thus investigated the CETA in relation to HDL concentration in a family with hyperalphalipoproteinemia (FHALP) [11]. Group I, FHALP persons had almost normal total cholesterol levels in comparison with their relatives (group II) and to a reference group (III), but very high HDL cholesterol values. The HDL cholesterol of one proband in group I was almost 5 mM.

Group I had a very low CETA if expressed in % cholesterol ester transfer/h, only 1.7%/h for the proband with the HDL cholesterol value of 5 mM. The probands of groups II and III had CETA values about 10 times higher.

Upon calculation of these results in terms of cholesterol exchange (in nmoles/ml/h) there was little difference between all three groups.

We also found a highly significant negative correlation between the cholesterol ester transfer rate and the concentration of HDL cholesterol. The higher the absolute concentration of HDL is, the lower the relative amount of CE transferred to VLDL and LDL. But the activity itself, the amount of enzyme, is probably high or not significantly different from normal lipemics.

Lp(a) as substrate of CETP

In another study we investigated Lp(a) with respect to its substrate properties for CETP.

The chemical composition as well as the structure of Lp(a) is very similar to LDL, but Lp(a) has a higher molecular weight. The core lipids of Lp(a) are identical with LDL; both are very rich in CE.

We studied the metabolism of Lp(a) and postulated on the basis of our results that Lp(a) has no TG-rich precursor. We believe that Lp(a) is secreted by the liver in its final form. Since the core lipids of Lp(a) and LDL are not much different, we were interested in the question whether Lp(a) obtains its CE by CETA [12].

After incubation of Lp(a) and LDL in the presence of HDL and purified CETP we found the reactivity of Lp(a) for CETP to be approx. 50% that of LDL. The removal of the Apo-(a)-protein, which is attached on the surface of Lp(a) via -S-S- bridge, by the addition of dithiothreitol or mercaptoethanol, yielded a particle which was free of Apo(a). This new particle resembled LDL chemically and structurally, and served as a substrate of CETP as good as LDL.

Conclusion

From the results of our studies, together with those of other laboratories, we conclude that LCAT plays an integral role in the overall metabolism of plasma lipoproteins. LCAT also, in concert with LPL, TG-rich lipoproteins, and CETP, is responsible for the structure and chemical composition of lipoproteins found in normal plasma. Nascent lipoproteins, VLDL, chylomicrons, and disk-shaped HDL are secreted from liver and intestine LPL hydrolyzes TG, leaving additional disk-like material, which is attacked by LCAT. The CE, which is synthesized during this reaction, gives rise to the formation of spherical HDL; CE are transfered to VLDL and LDL or exchanged by TG. TG-rich HDL, exhibiting most of the characteristics of HDL-2, are attacked by the liver lipase and rendered again into HDL-3.

LCAT plays also an important role in the LDL metabolism since it was found that the receptor pathway is modulated by this enzyme. Finally it is responsible, together with CETP, for the CE content in Lp(a), a lipoprotein of high atherogenicity.

References

1. Glomset JA (1973) Adv Lipid Res 11: 1–65
2. Hamilton RL, Williams MC, Fielding CJ, Havel RJ (1975) J Clin Invest 58: 3–10
3. Albers JJ, Tollefson JH, Chen CH, Steinmetz A (1984) Arteriosclerosis 4: 49–58
4. Fielding CJ, Shore VG, Fielding PE (1972) Biochem Biophys Res Commun 46: 1493–1498
5. Steyrer E, Kostner GM (1988) Biochim Biophys Acta 958: 484–491
6. Dieplinger H, Zechner R, Kostner GM (1985) J Lipid Res 26: 273–282
7. Zechner R, Dieplinger H, Roscher A, Kostner GM (1984) Biochem J 224: 569–576
8. Kostner GM, Krempler F, Dieplinger H, Zechner R, Teubl I, Sandhofer F (1985) Clin Sci 68: 411–418
9. Knipping G, Zechner R, Kostner GM, Holasek A (1985) Biochim Biophys Acta 835: 244–252
10. Knipping G, Birchbauer A, Steyrer E, Kostner GM (1987) Biochemistry 26: 7945–7953
11. Groener JEM, DaCol P, Kostner GM (1987) Biochem J 242: 27–32
12. Groener JEM, Kostner GM (1987) J Lipid Res 28: 1053–1056

Role of the Liver in the Metabolism of Lipoprotein Particles

A. Van Tol

Introduction

The liver is an important organ for lipoprotein metabolism. It is not only a major site of lipoprotein synthesis, but also the most important site of lipoprotein catabolism. Most of the apolipoproteins, as well as the cholesterol and cholesterylester moieties of all circulating plasma lipoproteins, are catabolized in the liver. This makes sense because the liver is the only organ capable of degrading substantial amounts of cholesterol. The resulting bile acids are secreted in the bile, together with undegraded cholesterol. A small part of the bile acids and cholesterol escapes the enterohepatic circulation and forms the major route of cholesterol excretion from the body.

The lipoproteins present in plasma may be operationally defined according to their density, as low or very low density lipoproteins and high density lipoproteins, but other, more functional definitions may be more appropriate in connection with in vivo metabolism. Examples are the lipoprotein classes chylomicrons and chylomicron remnants. Alaupovic has suggested a classification based on the apolipoprotein composition [1]. As apolipoproteins often determine the metabolic fate of lipoprotein particles this is a logical approach. Lipoprotein particles with specific apolipoprotein compositions exist in all density fractions of human plasma, as well as plasma from a variety of animal species.

It can be expected that all plasma lipoprotein classes, defined in one way or another, consist of a variety of subfractions, simply because plasma lipoproteins form a dynamic system. Plasma lipoprotein metabolism starts as soon as the nascent particles are secreted. Subsequent intravascular metabolism includes the actions of lipoprotein lipase, hepatic lipase, lecithin: cholesterol acyltransferase (LCAT), and lipid transfer proteins (LTP). In addition, most lipoproteins can bind to lipoprotein receptors. This can be followed by uptake and irreversible intracellular degradation of the holo-particle, or by reappearance in plasma of a modified form of the lipoprotein. The modifications may be due to the transfer of cellular lipids to plasma lipoproteins or to the specific transfer of lipoprotein components to the cells. Both mechanisms may include retroendocytosis.

Apolipoproteins as Determinants of Lipoprotein Metabolism

Data from the literature [1] were used to calculate (with some assumptions), the relative distribution of Apo B between the different Apo B-containing particles in

H. U. Klör (Ed.)
Lipoprotein Subfractions
Omega-3 Fatty Acids
© Springer-Verlag Berlin Heidelberg 1989

Table 1. Distribution of Apo B in Human Plasma Lipoproteins

	VLDL	IDL	LDL
Normals ($n = 8$)			
LP-B:C:E	63%	21%	9%
LP-B:C	15%	4%	3%
LP-B	22%	75%	88%
FH heterozygotes ($n = 3$)			
LP-B:C:E	34%	17%	10%
LP-B:C	11%	4%	–
LP-B	55%	79%	90%
Primary hyper TG ($n = 5$)			
LP-B:C:E	52%	25%	15%
LP-B:C	47%	20%	5%
LP-B	1%	55%	80%

human lipoprotein density fractions. Table 1 shows the relative amounts of Apo B in LP B:C:E, LP B:C and LP B in VLDL, IDL and LDL.

It is clear that the distributions may differ substantially between hypertrigly-ceridemic and hypercholesterolemic states. How may these apolipoprotein compositions influence metabolism? In order to answer this type of basic question it is often necessary to turn to animal experiments.

Yamada et al. [2] have separated Apo B-containing particles from rabbit plasma in B, E particles and B particles, by immunosorption on columns of anti-apolipoprotein E bound to Sepharose, and determined their distribution within the VLDL, IDL, and LDL density classes. After specific labelling of the Apo B moiety, it was possible to study separately the turnover rates of B, E particles and B particles. It was found that B, E particles in the VLDL density range are metabolized much faster than B particles. The difference between the catabolic rates of B, E particles and B particles from the IDL density range was much smaller and no clearcut difference between the in vivo decay rates of the two particle types was observed any longer when labelled particles from the LDL density range were injected.

Both Apo B and Apo B, E lipoproteins can be recognized and bound by the LDL or B-E receptor. One possible explanation for the more rapid metabolism of B, E particles from the VLDL density range compared with B, E particles from the IDL and LDL density range may be found in the differences in size. Particles with VLDL density generally are much bigger than particles from IDL and LDL. It was shown that the molar ratio of Apo E to Apo B varies with particle diameter and it can be calculated that the B, E particles in LDL will carry only a single Apo E molecule, while the large B, E particles from VLDL may carry three to four Apo E molecules. The rapid metabolism of VLDL remnants (B, E particles from the VLDL density range), observed by many investigators in a variety of animal species, may be caused by a polyvalent binding to the LDL receptor. The separation of lipoproteins according to size therefore gives important information, in addition to separations based on density or apolipoprotein composition. The possible role of a putative hepatic chylomicron remnant or Apo E receptor in VLDL-remnant metabolism needs further investigation.

Tissue Sites of Plasma (Very) Low Density Lipoprotein Catabolism

The quantitatively important role of the liver in the metabolism of labelled VLDL remnants or chylomicron remnants can be demonstrated quite easily in the rat, using conventionally iodinated lipoproteins or lipoproteins labelled biosynthetically with radioactive amino acids, e. g, 3-H-leucine. Groot et al. used the latter technique in a study of chylomicron remnant turnover [3]. The remnants have a very rapid turnover and the label, present on the Apo B moiety of chylomicron remnants, is almost quantitatively recovered in the liver within 15 min. In order to study in vivo catabolic sites of lipoproteins with slower turnover rates (LDL and HDL), or to study catabolic sites in animal species with slower metabolic rates than the rat, other experimental approaches must be taken. Using the model of partial hepatectomy, we showed that the liver is the most important organ removing injected homologous ^{125}I-LDL from rat plasma [4]. Removal of ⅔ of the liver resulted in a 60% decrease in the fractional catabolic rate of iodinated LDL, suggesting that the liver is by far the most important catabolic site of LDL. The synthesis of nondegradable labels provided a valuable improvement in the field of catabolic site studies. The rationale behind this "trapped ligand method" is that conventionally iodinated proteins are degraded without intracellular accumulation of their degradation products. Nondegradable labels, however, accumulate intracellularly, because of the presence of a sucrose, raffinose, or a cellobiose moiety. We used the diazo-iodobenzoylsucrose (DIBS) label [5]. Using various nondegradable labels it was shown that the liver is the most important site of LDL degradation in a variety of species. Its contribution to the total LDL turnover varies between 60% and 90%. The hepatic degradation of homologous LDL was found to be mostly receptor-dependent. On the contrary, in vivo degradation of human LDL in the rat is receptor-independent [5–9].

Bilheimer et al. described a very impressive experiment demonstrating the role of the liver in LDL degradation [10]. A combined liver-heart transplantation was performed as treatment for the homozygous form of familial hypercholesterolemia. After transplantation of the liver from a normal donor, the patient's extremely high plasma LDL-cholesterol level was normalized and her fractional catabolic rate of LDL increased several-fold.

Tissue Sites of High Density Lipoprotein Catabolism

The uptake by tissues and degradation of high density lipoproteins (HDL) is more complex than the metabolism of chylomicron remnants, IDL, or LDL. In contrast to lipoproteins of lower density, which are catabolized by receptor-mediated endocytosis of the holo-particle, animal experiments show that the lipid and apolipoprotein moieties of HDL are metabolized separately and often at different rates [11]. Table 2 summarizes our experiments in rats.

HDL was labelled either in the protein moiety or in the cholesterylester moiety and the rates of turnover were compared after intravenous injection. A biphasic serum decay was observed for the cholesterylester as well as the apolipoprotein moieties. Both the halflife ($t\frac{1}{2}$) of the second decay phase and the calculated fractional turnover rate (FTR) were significantly different. In the same type of experiments we observed

Table 2. Kinetic parameters of HDL turnover in the rat

	Apolipo-proteins	Cholesteryl-esters
t½ first phase (h)	0.3 ± 0.1	0.2 ± 0.1
t½ second phase (h)	6.2 ± 0.3	4.2 ± 0.4**
F.T.R. (day $^{-1}$)	2.9 ± 0.2	4.8 ± 0.2**

$P < 0.001$**

a significant effect of partial hepatectomy on the turnover of HDL cholesteryl-esters, but not on the turnover of HDL apolipoproteins A and C [11, 12]. At the time we were surprised by the absence of a significant effect of partial hepatectomy on the fractional catabolic rate of HDL apolipoprotein. Subsequently it became clear that the kidneys are very active in the degradation of HDL apolipoproteins A-I, A-IV and E [13, 14]. These and other experiments mitigated the role of the liver in HDL apolipoprotein degradation and stressed the hepatic role in HDL-cholesterylester uptake. Table 2 shows that the turnover of the HDL cholesterylesters in control animals is faster than that of HDL apolipoproteins. The HDL cholesterylesters are almost quantitatively taken up by the liver, while the protein moieties are partly degraded in the kidneys.

HDL consists of a variety of subfractions [15]. A difference in metabolic behavior between Apo E- and cholesterol-rich HDL and Apo A-rich HDL may explain part of the preferential uptake of the cholesterylesters in the liver. However, this phenomenon is also observed using Apo E-free HDL [16]. Using nondegradable lipid and protein labels it was shown not only that the in vivo clearance rate of cholesterylesters/ethers is higher, but also that the preferential uptake is not limited to the liver. It also occurs in steroid-producing tissues like the adrenals and ovaries [16]. These sites (liver, adrenals, ovaries) coincide with the presence of a heparin-releasable tissue lipase, different from lipoprotein lipase [17]. The role of this hepatic lipase in cholesterol metabolism is still not clear, but arguments in favour of a possible function in the preferential uptake of HDL cholesterylesters as well as HDL-unesterified cholesterol have been presented [18, 19].

Putative HDL receptors have been proposed in a variety of organs, including kidneys [20] and liver [21–23]. Table 3 shows that the specific binding of rat HDL to kidney membranes is not dependent on the Apo E content of HDL.

In contrast, HDL binding to liver membranes is very much dependent on the content of Apo E. Treatment of rats with 17-alpha-ethinylestradiol (EE) does not

Table 3. Specific binding of high density lipoproteins to partially purified liver and kidney membranes

	Liver		Kidney
	Control	17 α-EE	
Apo E-rich HDL	1.24	1.16	1.06 ± 0.15
Control HDL	0.62 ± 0.07	0.63 ± 0.10	0.96 ± 0.35
Apo E-poor HDL	0.22	0.34	1.18 ± 0.32

Values are given as µg HDL bound/mg membrane protein, measured with 25 µg HDL protein/ml at 0°C

increase the binding of HDL, despite the induction of LDL receptors. This shows that hepatic LDL receptors do not interact with typical (Apo E-containing) rat HDL [24]. These data indicate that the putative chylomicron remnant or Apo E receptor could be responsible for the binding of Apo E-containing rat HDL. A role of HDL or Apo A receptors in the hepatic metabolism of plasma HDL has not yet been firmly established. As mentioned before, HDL contains several subfractions. The most important lipoprotein particles in human HDL are LP-A-I and LP-A-I + A-II. The study of the interaction of these HDL subfractions with cultured Hep G2 cells is under investigation.

Intravascular Remodelling of Plasma Lipoproteins

The cholesterylesters present on plasma lipoproteins are partly secreted into the plasma on nascent lipoproteins (chylomicrons and VLDL) and partly synthesized by the plasma enzyme LCAT. In some species, including man, active lipid transfer proteins (LTP) circulate in plasma. Both LCAT and LTP are synthesized in the liver (for reviews, see [25, 26]). Cholesterylester transfer protein (CETP) catalyses a transfer/exchange of cholesterylesters between HDL and the other lipoproteins. This process is important for the turnover of plasma cholesterol because, depending on the amount of active CETP and the chemical composition of the circulating plasma lipoproteins, a variable part of the HDL-cholesterylesters are transferred by CETP to lipoprotein classes of lower density, or vice versa. The presence of active CETP seems to provide a link between VLDL/IDL/LDL metabolism on one hand, and HDL metabolism on the other. In addition LTP may directly influence the hepatic uptake of cholesterylesters from lipoproteins by as yet unknown mechanisms.

The distribution of plasma cholesterol between HDL, on one hand, and VLDL/IDL/LDL on the other, is strongly related to the prevalence of coronary heart disease. LTP are able to catalyse cholesterylester transport in either direction. Therefore, elucidation of the mechanism of action and regulation of lipid transfer processes should contribute to our understanding of atherogenesis.

References

1. Alaupovic P, Tavella M, Fesmire J (1987) Separation and identification of Apo-B-containing lipoprotein particles in normolipidemic subjects and patients with hyperlipoproteinemias. In: Advances in Experimental Biology and Medicine, Vol. 210, Malmendier CL, Alaupovic P (Eds), Lipoproteins and Atherosclerosis. Plenum, New York, pp 7–14
2. Yamada N, Shames DM, Stoudemire JB, Havel RJ (1986) Metabolism of lipoproteins containing apolipoprotein B 100 in blood plasma of rabbits: heterogeneity related to the presence of apolipoprotein E. Proc Natl Acad Sci USA 83: 3479–3483
3. Groot PHE, Van Berkel TJC, Van Tol A (1981) Relative contributions of parenchymal and non-parenchymal (sinusoidal) liver cells in the uptake of chylomicron remnants. Metabolism 30: 792–797
4. Van Tol A, Van't Hooft FM, Van Gent T (1978) Discrepancies in the catabolic pathways of rat and human low density lipoproteins as revealed by partial hepatectomy in the rat. Atherosclerosis 29: 449–457

5. Van't Hooft FM, Van Tol A (1985) Application of O-(4-diazo-3-[^{125}]iodobenzoyl) sucrose for the detection of the catabolic sites of low density lipoprotein. FEBS Lett 179: 225–228
6. Pittman RC, Steinberg D (1984) Sites and mechanisms of uptake and degradation of high density and low density lipoproteins. J Lipid Res 25: 1577–1585
7. Van't Hooft FM, Van Tol A (1985) In vivo catabolism of human low density lipoprotein in the rat is mediated by a nonsaturable, low-affinity mechanism. FEBS Lett 183: 138–142
8. Van't Hooft FM, Van Tol A (1985) The sites of degradation of purified rat low density lipoprotein and high density lipoprotein in the rat. Biochim Biophys Acta 836: 344–353
9. Spady DK, Meddings JB, Dietschy JM (1986) Kinetic constants for receptor dependent and receptor independent low density lipoprotein transport in the tissues of the rat and hamster. J Clin Invest 77: 1474–1481
10. Bilheimer DW, Goldstein JL, Grundy SM, Starzl TE, Brown MS (1984) Liver transplantation to provide low-density-lipoprotein receptors and lower plasma cholesterol in a child with homozygous familial hypercholesterolemia. N Engl J Med 311: 1658–1661
11. Van't Hooft FM, Van Gent T, Van Tol A (1981) Turnover and uptake by organs of radioactive serum high-density lipoprotein cholesteryl esters and phospholipids in the rat in vivo. Biochem J 196: 877–885
12. Van Tol A, Van Gent T, Van't Hooft FM, Vlaspolder F (1978) High density lipoprotein catabolism before and after partial hepatectomy. Atherosclerosis 29: 439–448
13. Van't Hooft FM, Van Tol A (1985) The sites of degradation of rat high-density-lipoprotein apolipoprotein E specifically labelled with O-(4-diazo-3-[^{125}I]iodobenzoyl) sucrose. Biochem J 226: 715–721
14. Dallinga-Thie GM, Van't Hooft FM, Van Tol A (1986) Tissue sites of degradation of high density lipoprotein apolipoprotein A-IV in rats. Arteriosclerosis 6: 277–284
15. Dallinga-Thie GM, Schneijderberg VLM, Van Tol A (1986) Identification and characterization of rat serum lipoprotein subclasses. Isolation by chromatography on agarose columns and sequential immunoprecipitation. J Lipid Res 27: 1035–1043
16. Pittman RC, Steinberg D (1986) A novel mechanism by which high density lipoprotein selectively delivers cholesterol esters to the liver. In: Receptor-mediated uptake in the liver. Greten H, Windler E, Beisiegel U (Eds). Springer, Berlin Heidelberg New York, pp 108–119
17. Jansen H, De Greef WJ (1981) Heparin-releasable lipase activity of rat adrenals, ovaries and testes. Biochem J 196: 739–745
18. Collet X, Perret B, Chollet F, Hullin F, Chap H, Douste-Blazy L (1988) Uptake of HDL unesterified and esterified cholesterol by human endothelial cells. Biochim Biophys Acta 958: 81–92
19. Bamberger M, Glick JM, Rothblat GH (1983) Hepatic lipase stimulates the uptake of high-density lipoprotein cholesterol by hepatoma cells. J Lipid Res 24: 869–876
20. Van Tol A, Dallinga-Thie GM, Van Gent T, Van't Hooft FM (1986) Specific saturable binding of rat high density lipoproteins to rat kidney membranes. Biochim Biophys Acta 876: 340–351
21. Fidge NH, Nestel PJ (1985) Identification of apolipoproteins involved in the interaction of human high density lipoproteins with receptors on cultured cells. J Biol Chem 260: 3570–3575
22. Rifici VA, Eder HA (1984) A hepatocyte receptor for high density lipoproteins specific for apolipoprotein A-I. J Biol Chem 259: 13814–13815
23. Graham DL, Oram JF (1987) Identification and characterization of a high density lipoprotein binding protein in cell membranes by ligand blotting. J Biol Chem 262: 7439–7442
24. Van't Hooft FM, Van Gent T, Van Tol A (1987) Effect of 17-alpha-ethinylestradiol on the catabolism of high-density lipoprotein apolipoprotein A-I in the rat. Atherosclerosis 67: 23–31
25. Fielding CJ (1987) Factors affecting the rate of catalysed transfer of cholesteryl esters in plasma. Amer Heart J 113: 532–537
26. Barter PJ, Hopkins GJ, Ha YC (1987) The role of lipid transfer proteins in plasma lipoprotein metabolism. Amer Heart J 113: 538–542

LDL Subfractions and Atherosclerosis

G. R. THOMPSON

To obtain subfractions LDL was first isolated in the conventional manner between density 1.019 and 1.063 and its density readjusted to 1.050. It was then sandwiched into the center of a five-step gradient as described by Teng et al. [1] and centrifuged in a swinging bucket SW 50.1 rotor for 40h at 10°C. At the end of the 40 h two clearly separated bands were visible towards the top of the tube, which were called light LDL and heavy LDL; under some circumstances a third band of heavier LDL is visible, but in most people one sees just two bands (Fig. 1). Using a Beckman fraction recovery system, it is possible to take off the gradient in 0.5-ml fractions, and thus recover these two fractions separately.

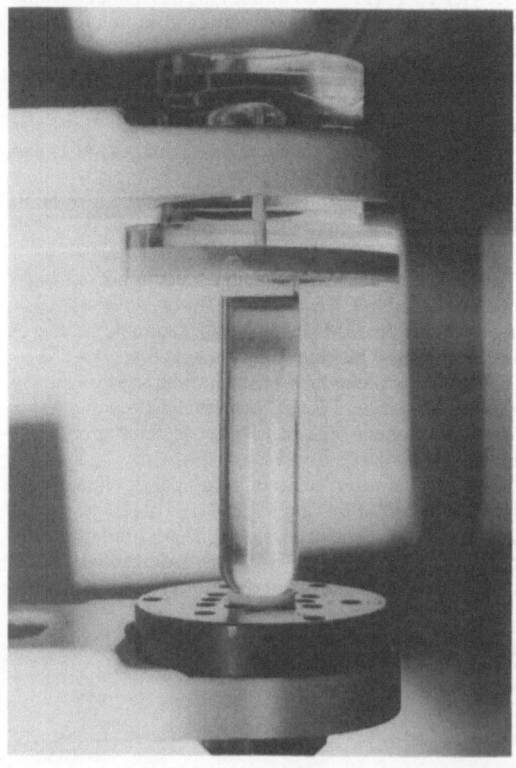

Fig. 1. Light *(upper)* and heavy *(lower)* subfractions of LDL after density-gradient ultracentrifugation

H. U. Klör (Ed.)
Lipoprotein Subfractions
Omega-3 Fatty Acids
© Springer-Verlag Berlin Heidelberg 1989

Studies of ApoB Metabolism

Some studies were carried out in three groups of subjects: control subjects, patients with hyperapobetalipoproteinemia (hyperapoB) and patients with heterozygous familial hypercholesterolemia (FH). The hyperapoB patients tended to be hypertriglyceridemic, whereas the FH patients were markedly hypercholesterolemic. LDL cholesterol was, by definition, normal in the controls, and in the hyperapoB group, but markedly elevated in FH patients. LDL-ApoB levels were normal in the controls, raised in the hyperapoB and even more markedly raised in the FH patients. Perhaps the most important point is that the cholesterol:ApoB ratio in LDL, which was slightly high in the FH patients, was conspicuously reduced in the hyperapoB subjects; this is very much a distinguishing feature of this syndrome. Turnover studies were performed on these three groups, injecting them with ^{125}I-labelled VLDL and ^{131}I-labelled LDL [2]. The controls and the FH patients had very similar rates of VLDL-ApoB synthesis, but synthesis was markedly elevated in hyperapoB subjects. The fractional catabolic rate (FCR) of both groups of patients was slightly reduced compared with controls, and since pool sizes reflect the combined effects of oversynthesis and reduced catabolism, the VLDL pool was appreciably bigger in the hyperapoB patients than in the two other groups.

With respect to LDL turnover, there was a normal rate of LDL-ApoB synthesis in the control subjects, their FCR averaged 0.36/day and their pool size was just under 3 g. HyperapoB patients oversynthesised LDL-ApoB at about the same rate as the FH patients, but unlike the latter there was no reduction of FCR in hyperapoB, which was, if anything, slightly higher than in the control subjects. So that, in turnover terms, the hyperapoB and the FH patients both had increased rates of LDL-ApoB synthesis; in hyperapoB, this seems to be mainly on the basis of oversynthesis of VLDL, whereas direct synthesis of LDL is prominent in FH patients. Another difference was that the hyperapoB patients catabolized their LDL at a normal rate, whereas FH patients did not.

Looking at the subfractions, there was found out that in the control subjects about 60% of the ApoB carried in LDL was present in the heavy fraction, and in the remaining 40% it was in the light fraction. In hyperapoB patients, a slightly greater proportion was carried in the heavy fraction than in the control subjects, whereas in the FH patients, roughly equal amounts of ApoB were present in each of the two main subfractions.

In addition, there were differences in the cholesterol:ApoB ratio of subfractions. Under normal circumstances the heavy fraction has a slightly lower cholesterol:ApoB ratio than the light, this difference being exaggerated in hyperapoB; this is presumably the reason why whole LDL in this syndrome has such a low cholesterol:apoB ratio. In contrast, in FH there is an increase in cholesterol:ApoB ratio of the light subfraction. As regards size, light LDL normally has a slightly larger diameter than heavy LDL. In hyperapoB the heavy LDL tends to be smaller than normal and there is a tendency for the light LDL in FH to be larger than normal.

Interconversion of LDL Subfractions

Further turnover studies were done to try to work out the relationship between the light and heavy subfractions, by injecting them separately [3]. In essence, it appeared that light LDL was mainly produced as a result of the catabolism of VLDL via IDL and that normally most of the light LDL was then converted into heavy LDL, which is the main form in which LDL is irreversibly catabolized. But under certain circumstances there does seem to be some direct input of heavy LDL, which is independent of the normal VLDL/IDL pathway, and although most of the light LDL is converted into heavy LDL, some light LDL is irreversibly catabolized. Looking at the percentage of light LDL that was converted to heavy LDL in a small number of patients from each of these three groups, there was found out that in control subjects about 75% of the light LDL was converted to heavy LDL within the space of 2 weeks following the injection of labelled light LDL. If anything, a slightly higher proportion of light LDL was converted to heavy LDL in hyperapoB, whereas in FH there was a marked reduction in the proportion of light LDL that was converted into heavy LDL (Table 1). This presumably is one reason for the relative increase and accumulation of light LDL in FH patients.

Table 1. Deconvolution analysis of simultaneous turnovers of ^{125}I-L-LDL and ^{131}I-H-LDL

	% L → H
Control ($n = 2$)	74.7
HyperapoB ($n = 2$)	88.9
FH ($n = 4$)	57.4

Because the mechanism of the transformation from light into heavy LDL is not known, one can only speculate about this. Figure 2 shows a light LDL particle, and adjacent to it in the space of Disse of the liver, are VLDL particles. It has been shown by many workers that there is movement of cholesterol ester from LDL into VLDL, with reverse movement of triglyceride from VLDL back into LDL. One can envisage conversion of light into heavy LDL as reflecting movement of cholesterol ester out of light LDL accompanied by lipolysis of any triglyceride which it acquires in exchange. The net result is a slightly smaller LDL particle because it has less cholesterol ester per mole of protein. In hyperapoB patients, there is an excess of VLDL particles with a very rapid rate of flux and it may well be that exchange of cholesterol ester for triglyceride is accentuated, giving rise to even smaller heavy LDL particles than normal. Exactly what the role of the LDL receptor is in this process is not clear, but the fact that this transformation seems to be defective or slow in patients with FH would suggest that the LDL receptor plays either a direct or indirect role in this transformation. It is possible that hepatic lipase is also an important determinant of the normal conversion of light into heavy LDL, by mediating hydrolysis of LDL triglyceride.

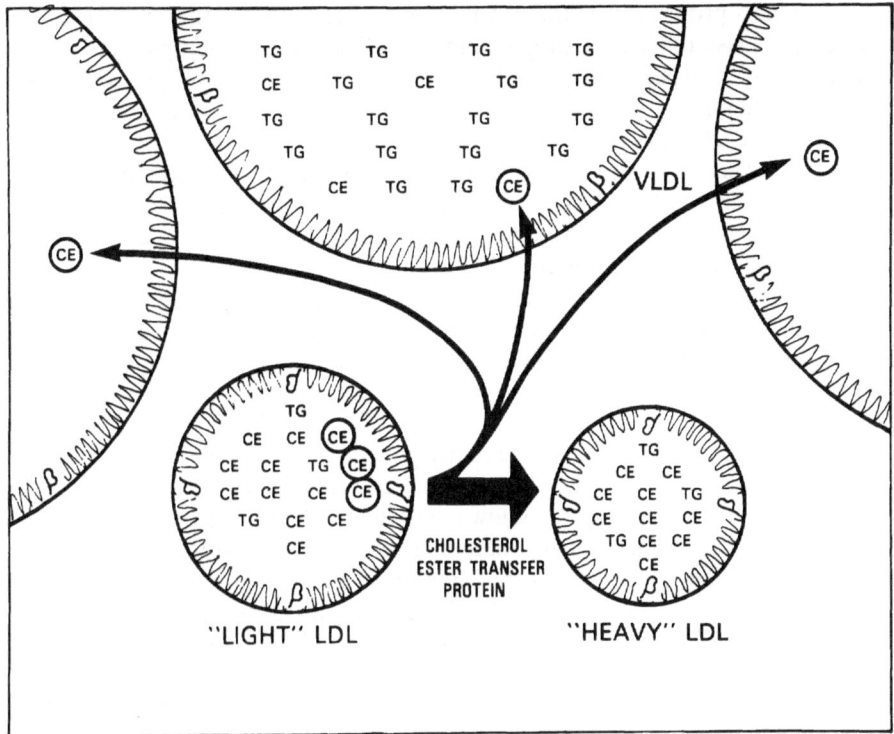

Fig. 2. Possible mechanism for conversion of light into heavy LDL, showing transfer of cholesterol ester (CE) from core of light LDL to adjacent VLDL particles

Atherogenic Role of LDL Subfractions

In relation to atherosclerosis, it is known that light LDL is atherogenic, as exemplified by FH homozygotes who get a peculiar form of athersclerosis involving the valves and supravalvular region of the aorta and the coronary ostia. It may be that these features reflect the known tendency for very high concentrations of LDL to aggregate when mechanically agitated, since these are the areas of maximum turbulence in the aorta.

Heterozygotes also show a considerable degree of athersclerosis, which again is attributable to high concentrations of light LDL in plasma. By the age of 30 a significant proportion of male and a lesser proportion of female heterozygotes will have coronary disease and this percentage increases with age. It must be pointed out that the type of coronary disease seen in heterozygotes, is less atypical than in homozygotes, but nevertheless does differ to some extent from other forms of atherosclerosis. This is illustrated by a study which was done a few years ago, where patients with heterozygous FH were looked at and compared with normocholesterolemic smokers [4]. It was found that 72% of the FH patients had triple-vessel disease, compared with only 16% of the normocholesterolemic smokers. Also the location of the disease differed in that FH patients had mainly a combination of proximal and distal lesions, whereas in the smokers many of the lesions were purely distal. It seems probable that the distribution and severity of athersclerosis in FH heterozygotes also reflects the preponderance of light LDL in their plasma.

With regard to hyperapoB and atherosclerosis, Sniderman et al. [5] have shown that when patients with coronary disease were divided into two groups according to whether their LDL cholesterol was below or above 200 mg/dl, many of those in the latter category had raised LDL-ApoB levels, i. e. hyperapoB. The latter disorder has many features in common with familial combined hyperlipidemia (FCH) and it is possible that they are one and the same entity. For example, Brunzell et al. [6] showed that six out of seven FCH patients they studied had a raised LDL-ApoB. If one compares such individuals, as they did, with others with familial hypertriglyceridemia it is apparent that the tendency to develop coronary disease is much higher in FCH [7]. Furthermore, the data of Goldstein et al. [8] suggest that familial combined hyperlipidemia is the most common form of genetically determined hyperlipidemia in patients with coronary disease.

How can it be reconciled that apparently patients in whom there is an excess of heavy LDL (as in FCH) are almost as susceptible to athersclerosis as patients with an excess of light LDL (as in FH)? It is known that when LDL penetrates the arterial wall it must be taken up by macrophages before an atherosclerotic lesion can develop. It seems that interaction with glycosaminoglycans in the arterial wall is important in determining the fate of intramural LDL, either by modifying it in such a way that it is taken up by macrophages or perhaps irreversibly binding it. Although each heavy LDL particle does not carry as much cholesterol as a light LDL particle, nevertheless, it is likely that it penetrates the intima more easily. Stender and Ziversmit [9] correlated intimal clearance, a measure of influx, against particle diameter and found that the lowest rate of influx occurred with VLDL, intermediate with LDL and highest with HDL. Although they did not subfractionate LDL it seems reasonable to presume that smaller LDL particles would have a higher rate of influx than larger particles. It must be kept in mind that heavy LDL in hyperapoB patients is appreciably smaller than normal heavy LDL and is quite a bit smaller than light LDL. These data provide a reasonable basis for explaining why both LDL subfractions appear to be atherogenic.

References

1. Teng B, Thompson GR, Sniderman AD, Forte TM, Krauss RM, Kwiterovich PO (1983) Composition and distribution of low density lipoprotein fractions in hyperapobetalipoproteinemia, normolipidemia and familial hypercholesterolemia. Proc Natl Acad Sci USA 80: 6662–6666
2. Teng B, Sniderman AD, Soutar AK, Thompson GR (1986) Metabolic basis of hyperapobetalipoproteinemia. Turnover of apolipoprotein B in low density lipoprotein and its precursors and subfractions compared with normal and familial hypercholesterolemia. J Clin Invest 77: 663–672
3. Thompson GR, Teng B, Sniderman AD, Kinetics of LDL subfractions. Am Heart J 113: 514–517
4. Sugrue DD, Thompson GR, Oakley CM, Trayner IM, Steiner RE (1981) Contrasting patterns of coronary atherosclerosis in normocholesterolemic smokers and patients with familial hypercholesterolemia. Br Med J 283: 1358–1360
5. Sniderman A, Shapiro S, Marpole D, Skinner B, Teng B, Kwiterovich PO (1980) Association of coronary atherosclerosis with hyperapobetalipoproteinemia [increased protein but normal cholesterol levels in human low density (β) lipoproteins]. Proc Natl Acad Sci USA 77: 604–608

6. Brunzell JD, Albers JJ, Chait A, Grundy SM, Groszek E, McDonald GB (1983) Plasma lipoproteins in familial combined hyperlipidemia and monogenic familial hypertriglyceridemia. J Lipid Res 24: 147–155
7. Brunzell JD, Schrott HG, Motulsky AG, Bierman EL (1976) Myocardial infarction in the familial forms of hypertriglyceridemia. Metabolism 25: 313–320
8. Goldstein JL, Schrott HG, Hazzard WR, Bierman EL, Motulsky AG (1973) Hyperlipidemia in coronary heart disease. II. Genetic analysis of lipid levels in 176 families and delineation of a new inherited disorder, combined hyperlipidemia. J Clin Invest 52: 1544–1568
9. Stender S, Zilversmit DB (1981) Transfer of plasma lipoprotein components and of plasma proteins into aortas of cholesterol-fed rabbits. Molecular size as a determinant of plasma lipoprotein influx. Arteriosclerosis 1: 38–49

HDL Subclasses and Atherosclerosis

P. Avogaro

The studies relating HDL to the prediction of IHD belong to two separate time periods. In a first period there are the pioneer studies by Barr et al. [1], Gofman et al. [2], and Nikkila [3]. The second period starts with the report of Miller and Miller [4]. Since then a large amount of data have stressed the inverse relationship existing between the level of HDL and the prevalence of ischemic heart disease (IHD) [5, 6].

HDL and Triglycerides: A Confounding Relationship

Some doubts have been raised, however, concerning the validity of this relationship. The first doubt comes from Gofman himself. It is not possible, according to Gofman, to conclude whether or not the observed lowering of HDL_2 and HDL_3 in ischemic heart disease is in excess of that anticipated from the inverse correlation existing between the two subclasses and the levels of lipoproteins with Sf 0-400. The same opinion has been shared by Robinson et al. [7], who observed that total HDL and HDL_2 are inversely related to a coronary risk score, including cigarette consumption, body mass index, serum triglycerides, physical activity, and alcohol consumption, whereas HDL_3 show no significant correlation. None of the HDL measurements, however, correlated significantly with risk score after allowing for the effect of triglycerides. The same conclusion was reached by Shaper et al. [8], who used a multivariate analysis in a prospective study of 7735 middle-aged men. Some studies, however, failed to assess the existence of the inverse relationship, claiming that the two parameters constitute two independent variables. Witzum et al. [9] studied a series of patients showing abnormally high levels of plasma triglycerides. Extensive manipulations including different diets, physical exercise, alcohol withdrawal, and treatment with clofibrate, succeeded in reducing the triglyceride levels but failed to normalize the low levels of HDL cholesterol, despite a baseline inverse relationship existing between the two parameters. The same dissociation has been recorded, after diet, in people with type I and type V hyperlipemia [10–12], and in type II treated with bile sequestrants [13]. It appears, therefore, that the inverse correlation between VLDL-TG and HDL-C is not a rule. In some patients who fail to normalize when TG decrease, two independent associate variables may occur simultaneously. There are no longitudinal data providing information about the level of risk in this peculiar category.

H. U. Klör (Ed.)
Lipoprotein Subfractions
Omega-3 Fatty Acids
© Springer-Verlag Berlin Heidelberg 1989

Are HDL$_2$ and/or HDL$_3$ Predictors or Discriminators of IHD?

Apparently according to Miller and Miller [4], there is a large consensus that HDL are an "anti-risk" factor. The clinical, epidemiological, and experimental data supporting this hypothesis have been already cited [1–4, 14–17]. Despite the huge amount of data in favour, however, two main questions remain "open":
1. Are the HDLs an independent predictive anti-risk or discriminator factor?
2. If the HDLs are protective, are HDL$_2$ and HDL$_3$ similarly protective?

Concerning the first question, we have already cited the opinions of Gofman et al. [2] and Robinson et al. [7]. According to them none of the HDL measurements correlate significantly with the risk score after allowing for the effect of triglycerides. They do not recommend the inclusion of HDL subfractions as routine screening tests for heart disease, even while they do not deny that, despite a lack of independence, total HDL remains a useful summary indicator of CHD risk. More recently, in a prospective study on the power of lipoprotein mass concentrations a predictors of progression of CHD, during a 5-year period it was observed that HDL$_2$ and HDL$_3$ subfractions do not differ significantly between men with and without definite progression of CHD [14]. Some excellent studies, therefore, do not support the hypothesis of HDL as an independent discriminator and/or predictor of IHD.

HDLs are a heterogeneous group of molecules in terms of density, flotation rate, protein-lipid composition [18]. Two main subclasses are usually referred to as HDL$_2$ and HDL$_3$. Anderson et al. [19] have stressed that the HDL$_2$ constitute the main bulk of HDL; they are responsible for the protective effect as well for the different prevalence of IHD in the two sexes, whereas HDL$_3$ are more mobile, less protective, and more dependent on environmental factors. The major contributions on the anti-risk effect of HDL substantially agree that HDL$_2$ exerts the major protective role and that it is significantly reduced in IHD, whereas HDL$_3$ is mostly normal [19].

Another consensus on the predominant role of HDL$_2$ comes from the study by Vergani and Bettale [20]. They have described a family overrepresented by IHD, in which a condition of hypoalphalipoproteinemia was the only biochemically abnormal trait. In the affected members there was a decrease of HDL-C, ApoA-I, and ApoA-II, while all the other components were normal. From a rate zonal UC analysis it was observed that peak HDL$_2$ was completely absent, whereas HDL$_3$ was present normally.

Only two studies have recorded an involvement of both HDL$_2$ and HDL$_3$ as discriminators and/or predictors of IHD. Gofman et al. [2] reported a significant decrease of HDL$_3$ in survivors of myocardial infarction (MI) even if less significant than the decrease shown by HDL$_2$. We too have observed in a UC study of MI survivors a significant decrease of both HDL$_2$ and HDL$_3$ concomitant with a significant increase of IDL and LDL [21].

Apolipoproteins of HDL (ApoA-I and ApoA-II)

HDL contain several apolipoproteins. They are ApoA-I, ApoA-II, ApoC, and ApoE. Apoproteins A-I and A-II are the most abundant, the amount of ApoA-I being relatively higher in HDL_2, whereas ApoA-II is largely confined to HDL_3. The two minor apolipoproteins associate preferentially with HDL_3 and shuttle between HDL_3 and VLDL. ApoA-I is the activator of LCAT, whereas ApoA-II primarily maintains the structural integrity of HDL; ApoC accumulates in HDL as a reservoir for transfer to VLDL, while ApoE interacts with high-affinity receptors in liver and peripheral tissues [22].

Studies performed on the behavior of apolipoproteins of HDL in IHD support the predominant role of HDL_2. Albers et al. [23] and Avogaro et al. [21, 24] showed that ApoA-I levels were reduced in MI survivors. These records were lately confirmed [25, 26], although not by Pilgen et al. [27], who found more significant variations of ApoA-II than ApoA-I.

Recently according to a new classification of HDL apoproteins, it has been observed that in coronary patients there is a decrease of Lp-A-I (lipoproteins that contain Apo-A-I, but not Apo-A-II), whereas Lp-A-I:A-II (lipoproteins that contain bot apoA-I and A-II) are normal [28]. A possible predictive role for ApoA-I is supported by the paper of Ishinawa et al. [29], which shows that the levels of ApoA-I are lower in people who have lately complained of IHD.

Little information is available on plasma concentrations of ApoE, although normal values of total plasma ApoE have been recorded in angiographically proven IHD [30, 31]. We have recorded normal amounts of total plasma ApoE in normolipidemic MI survivors, whereas HDL-E and the ratio HDL-E/ApoA-I were lower in patients than in controls [32]. It is likely that the reduced amount of HDL-E impairs "reverse" cholesterol transport [33].

References

1. Barr DP, Russ EM, Eder HA (1951) Protein-lipid relationship in human plasma: II. In Athero-sclerosis and related conditions. Am J Med 11: 480–484
2. Gofman JW, Young W, Tandy R (1966) Ischemic heart disease, atherosclerosis and longevity. Circulation 34: 679–697
3. Nikkila E (1953) Studies on the lipid protein relationship in normal and pathological sera and the effect of heparin on serum lipoproteins. Scand J Clin Lab Invest 5 [Suppl 8] 1–101
4. Miller CJ, Miller NE (1975) Plasma high density lipoprotein concentration and development of ischaemic heart disease. Lancet i: 16–19
5. Gotto AM, Miller NE, Oliver MF (1978) High density lipoproteins and atherosclerosis. Elsevier, Amsterdam
6. Miller NE, Miller GJ (1984) Clinical and metabolic aspects of high-density lipoproteins. Elsevier, Amsterdam
7. Robinson G, Ferns GAA, Bevan EA, Stocks J, Williams PT, Galton DJ (1987) High density lipoprotein subfractions and coronary risk factors in normal men. Atherosclerosis 7: 341–346
8. Shaper AG, Pocock SJ, Walker M, Phillips AN, Whitehead TP, MacFarlane PW (1985) Risk factors for ischaemic heart disease; the prospective phase of the british regional heart study. J Epidemiol Community Health 39: 197–209
9. Witztum JL, Dillingham MA, Glese W, Bateman J, Diekman C, Kammeyer-Blaufuss E, Wiedman S, Schonfeld G (1980) Normalization of triglycerides in type IV hyperlipoproteinemia fails to correct low levels of high-density-lipoprotein cholesterol. N Engl J Med 303: 907–914
10. Falko JM, Witztum JL, Schonfeld G, Bateman J (1979) Dietary treatment of type V hyperlipo-proteinemia fails to normalize low levels of high-density lipoprotein cholesterol. Ann Intern Med 91: 750–751

11. Herbert PN, Henderson LO (1979) Plasma triglycerides do not regulate high-density lipoprotein concentrations. Lancet i: 1368–1370
12. Manzato E, Baggio G, Zambon S, Previato L (1987) High density lipoproteins in hypertrigly-ceridemia. In: Catapano AL, Salvioli G, Vergani C (eds) High density lipoproteins; physiopathological aspects and clinical significance. Raven New York, p 161 (Atherosol rev, vol 16)
13. Witztum JL, Schonfeld G, Weidman SW (1976) The effects of cholestipol on the metabolism of very low density lipoproteins in man. J Lab Clin Med 88: 1008–1018
14. Miller GJ (1984) Epidemiological and chemical aspects of high-density lipoproteins. In: Miller NE, Miller GJ (eds) Clinical and metabolic aspects of high density lipoproteins. Elsevier, Amsterdam
15. Kannel WB, Castelli WP (1979) Is the serum total cholesterol an anachronism? Lancet ii: 950–951
16. Glueck CJ, Fallat RW, Millet F, Steiner PM (1975) Familial hyperalphalipoproteinemia. Arch Intern Med 136: 1025–1028
17. Avogaro P, Cazzolato G (1975) Familial hyper-HDL (α)-cholesterolemia. Atherosclerosis 22: 63–67
18. Bittolo Bon G, Cazzolato G, Avogaro P (1981) Preparative isotachophoresis of human high density lipoproteins HDL$_2$ and HDL$_3$. J Lipid Res 22: 998–1002
19. Anderson DW, Nichols AV, Pan SS, Lindgren FT (1978) High density lipoprotein distribution. Resolution and determination of three major components in a normal population sample. Atherosclerosis 29: 161–179
20. Vergani C, Bettale G (1981) Familial hypo-alpha-lipo-proteinaemia. Clin Chim Acta 114: 45–52
21. Avogaro P, Bittolo Bon G, Cazzolato G, Quinci GB, Belussi F (1978) Plasma levels of apolipoprotein A-I and apolipoprotein B in human atherosclerosis. Artery 4: 385–394
22. Mahley RW (1978) Alterations in plasma lipoproteins induced by cholesterol feeding in animals including man. In: Dietschy JM, Gotto AM, Outko JH (eds) Disturbances in lipid and lipoprotein metabolism. Am Physiol Soc, Bethesda, pp 181–197
23. Albers JJ, Wahl PW, Cabana GV, Hazzard WR, Hoover JJ (1976) Quantitation of apolipoprotein A-I of human plasma high density lipoprotein. Metabolism 25: 633–644
24. Avogaro P, Bittolo Bon G, Cazzolato G, Quinci GB (1979) Are apolipoproteins better discriminators than lipids for atherosclerosis? Lancet i: 901–903
25. Kladetzky RG, Assmann G, Walgenbach S, Tauchert P, Helb HD (1980) Lipoprotein and apoprotein values in coronary angiography patients. Artery 7: 191–195
26. Riesen W, Mordasini R, Salzmann C, Gurtner HP (1982) Apoproteins in angiographically documented coronary heart disease. In: Noseda C, Fragiacomo C, Fumagalli R, Paoletti R (eds) Lipoproteins and coronary atherosclerosis. Elsevier, Amsterdam, p 129
27. Pilgen E, Pristantz A, Pfeiffer KP, Kostner G (1983) Risk factors for peripheral atherosclerosis: retrospective evaluation by stepwise discriminant analysis. Arteriosclerosis 3: 57–63
28. Parra H, Fievet C, Boniface B, Bertrand M, Moschetto J, Fruchart JC (1984) Lipoproteins, apolipoproteins and coronary artery disease assessed by coronary arteriography. In: De Gennes JL et al. (eds) Latent and dyslipoproteinemias and atherosclerosis. Raven, New York, pp 87–197
29. Ishikawa T, Fidge N, Thelle DS, Forde OH, Miller NE (1978) The Tromso Heart Study: serum apolipoprotein A-I concentration in relation to future coronary heart disease. Eur J Clin Invest 8: 179–182
30. Tan MH, Weldon KL, Albers JJ, Cheung MC, Havel RJ, Vigne JL (1980) Serum HDL-cholesterol, ApoA-I and ApoE levels in patients with abnormal coronary arteries. Clin Invest Med 3: 225
31. Miller NE, Hammett F, Saltissi S, Rao S, Zeller HV, Coltart J, Lewis B (1981) Relation of angiographically defined coronary artery disease to plasma lipoprotein subfractions and apolipoproteins. Br Med J [Clin Res] 182: 1741
32. Bittolo Bon G, Cazzolato G, Saccardi M, Kostner GM, Avogaro P (1984) Total plasma ApoE and high density lipoprotein ApoE in survivors of myocardial infarction. Atherosclerosis 53: 69–75
33. Mahley RW (1981) Cellular and molecular biology of lipoprotein metabolism in atherosclerosis. Diabetes 30 [Suppl 2]: 60

Lipoprotein Deficiency Syndromes

C. R. SIRTORI

Introduction

Deficiency of mature lipoprotein fractions, be it the consequence of an abnormality of the apolipoprotein(s) or of a deficient synthesis, can have a significant clinical impact in some cases whereas in others it may go almost unnoticed. The study of lipoprotein deficiency syndromes has received considerable help from the recent advances in molecular cloning both of apolipoproteins and of major enzymes involved in lipid metabolism. This type of information has allowed the conclusion that lipoprotein deficiency syndromes are very often associated with well-characterized abnormalities in the processing and/or transformation of lipoproteins or apolipoproteins in the carriers.

Apolipoprotein B Deficiency

A betalipoproteinemia was first described by Bassen and Kornzweig [3], and was associated with retinitis pigmentosa, erythrocyte abnormalities, and mental retardation. It is transmitted as an autosomal recessive trait. Homozygous patients are characterized by virtually complete absence of both forms of Apo B, Apo B-100 and Apo B-48, as well as of the Apo B-containing lipoproteins: chylomicrons, very low density lipoproteins (VLDL), and low density lipoproteins (LDL) [22]. Heterozygous subjects are essentially normal.

Hypobetalipoproteinemia is also characterized by plasma Apo B deficiency in the homozygous state, but Apo B levels are also reduced distinctly in obligate heterozygotes [22]. Most interesting is a third variant of Apo B deficiency, *normotriglyceridemic abetalipoproteinemia,* characterized by the presence in plasma of Apo B-48 but not of Apo B-100 [21].

Patients with this condition (Table 1) show a typical hypolipidemia, with only a slight postprandial rise, and almost complete deficiency of LDL. Apo B-100 is clearly absent in the plasma of this patient in Fig. 1 whereas Apo B-48 is evident in chylomicrons.

The biochemical defect in abetalipoproteinemic patients has been recently investigated by gene expression in leukocytes and liver cells [18]. Interestingly, polyadenylated hepatic Apo B-100 messenger ribonucleic acid (mRNA) is normally expressed, levels being increased sixfold in comparison with control hepatic Apo B-100 mRNA levels. These findings are consistent with a posttranslational error in Apo B processing or secretion.

H. U. Klör (Ed.)
Lipoprotein Subfractions
Omega-3 Fatty Acids
© Springer-Verlag Berlin Heidelberg 1989

Table 1. Biochemical characteristics of Apo-B 100 deficiency

Plasma cholesterol (mg/dl)	25
Plasma triglyceride (mg/dl)	30
postprandial	200
Postprandial lipoproteins (mg/dl)	
$d < 1.006$	96
$1.006 < d < 1.063$	1
$1.063 < d < 1.210$	74

From [21]

d, Relative density

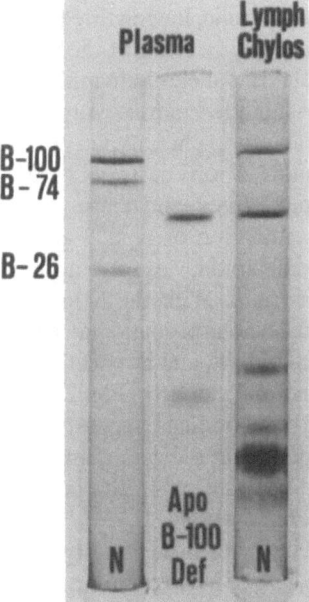

Fig. 1. Apolipoproteins from low-density lipoproteins of a normal *(N)* and from an Apo B-100 deficient subject, compared with chylomicrons of a normal individual. SDS electrophoreses were carried out in 3% polyacrylamide gels. It is clearly apparent that in LDL of the Apo B-100 deficient subject no Apo B-100 can be found, whereas the only apolipoprotein has an identical mobility to Apo B-48 [21]

Recently, the originally defined "normotriglyceridemic hypobetalipoproteinemia" [36] was reinvestigated in the original kindred. An abnormal Apo B species, Apo B-37 (203 kd), was found by SDS electrophoretic separation in several members of the kindred. The Apo B-37 variant, detectable both in VLDL and in high-density lipoproteins (HDL) by immunochemical analyses, contains only the amino-terminal domain of Apo B-100. The most remarkable feature of Apo B-37 is that it is prevalent in the HDL density region within discrete lipoprotein B-37 particles [39]. These findings suggest a complex metabolic alteration in the carriers but, in spite of this, clinical effects are minimal. Examination of 41 family members in 3 generations showed the presence of two mutant Apo B alleles associated with low Apo B and LDL-cholesterol levels [39]. One allele results in the production of the truncated B-37, with LDL-cholesterol at around 6 mg/dl and mild fat malabsorption, and the other in reduced Apo B-100 and LDL-cholesterol (31 ± 15 mg/dl).

In conclusion, it appears that Apo B deficiency, when clinically pronounced, may be accompanied by red cell alterations, heredoataxia, and malabsorption. However, in heterozygotes and in carriers of Apo B-37, symptoms may be minimal. The neurological syndrome as well as the retinal degeneration in abetalipoproteinemic patients may be partially sensitive to vitamin E supplementation [24].

Apolipoprotein E Deficiency

Apo E, a quantitatively minor apolipoprotein, is a 34-kd glycoprotein constituent of plasma triglyceride-rich lipoproteins and of HDL. The functional role of Apo E is most likely that of interaction with the remnant receptor in the liver [26]. Apo E is polymorphic, having three major isoforms separated by isoelectric focusing (Apo E2, E3, and E4). Each of the three polymorphic forms of Apo E is coded by a separate allele; the alleles being inherited in a codominant fashion at a single genetic locus.

A unique kindred with premature cardiovascular disease, tuberoeruptive xanthomas, and, phenotypically, a type III hyperlipoproteinemia, was found to have familial Apo E deficiency [13]. VLDL were markedly enriched in cholesterol in the homozygotes, and these same patients had only minimal amounts of Apo E, with accumulation of Apo B-48 and Apo A-IV in VLDL and LDL. In heterozygotes, plasma lipid levels were normal with mean plasma Apo E concentrations about 42% of normal. With the help of turnover studies it has been possible to show that a homozygous proband had a marked delay in the fractional catabolism of VLDL Apo B-100, B-48, and E, together with an extremely low Apo E synthetic rate, compared to normal subjects (Fig. 2) [31].

These findings suggest that deficiency of Apo E is responsible for an overall reduction in the catabolism of VLDL, thus leading to an enrichment with Apo B-48 and cholesterol. In the homozygous condition this may be accompanied by severe arterial disease.

The mechanism underlying the reduced synthesis of Apo E has been examined with the help of in vitro studies on macrophages, comparing the expression of Apo E from normals and Apo E-deficient subjects. These studies clearly show an extreme reduction of mRNA in the Apo E-deficient condition [1].

The molecular defect has recently been linked [7] to a single base substitution, an A→G transversion, in the penultimate 3' nucleotide of the third intron of the Apo E gene. This leads to a loss of the correct 3' splice site, thus giving rise to two abnormally spliced mRNA forms. The smaller form contains 53 nucleotides and the larger one, the entire third intron of the gene. Since both mRNA species contain chain termination codons within the intronic sequence, only short Apo E peptides not detectable by standard gel electrophoretic techniques are produced. Apo E deficiency is, therefore, the result of a molecular error which gives rise to shorter, nonfunctional forms of Apo E. In contrast to Apo B, where the mechanism is posttranslational, here it is clearly pretranslational.

Apolipoprotein C-II Deficiency

Apo C-II is the apolipoprotein responsible for the normal catabolism of VLDL. It is capable of interacting both with the capillary wall and with the lipoprotein particles,

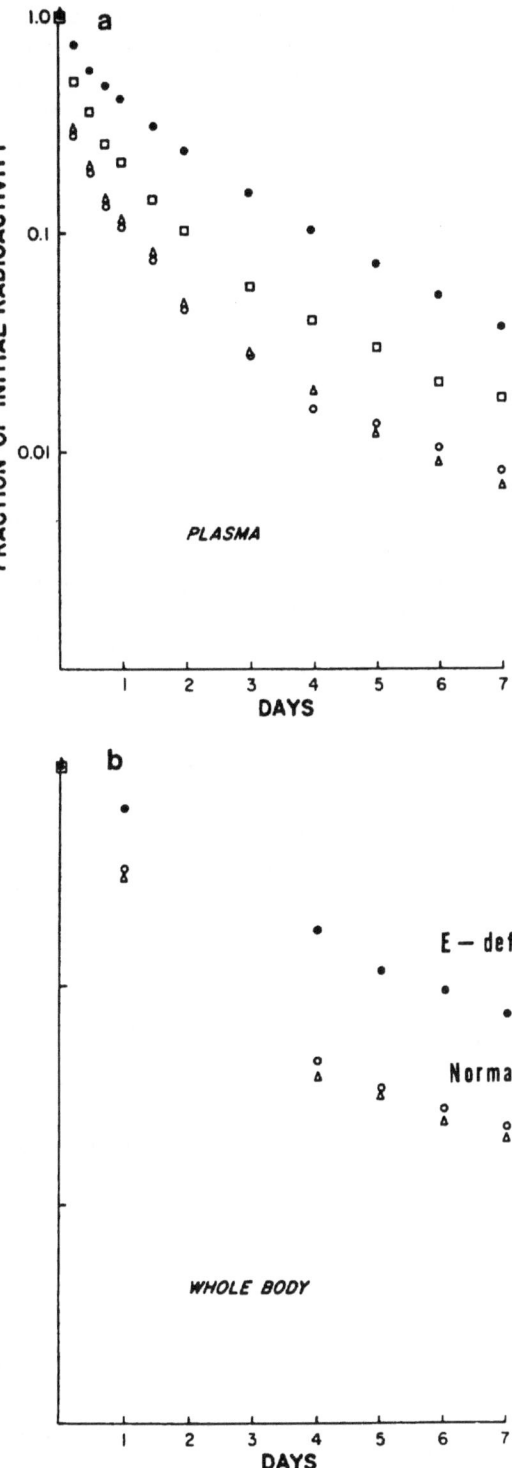

Fig. 2a, b. Plasma turnover of labeled apolipoprotein E in normals *(open symbols)* and in an E-deficient patient *(filled circles)*. Considerably slower turnover is noted in the latter [29]

thus acting as a protease and as a co-lipase [15]. About 10 years ago, the first case of so-called "Apo C-II deficiency" was reported in Canada [4]. At that time methods of analysis lacked sophistication and it was generally accepted on the basis of results using plain SDS gels that there was evidence of C-II deficiency. These patients showed severe hypertriglyceridemia. Similarly, C-II deficiencies were described in Padova [2], Bethesda, etc.

Serious doubt was cast on the hypothesis of a simple Apo C-II deficiency by the observation [19] that if a C-II immunoblot is carried out on isoelectric focusing gels of VLDL from C-II-deficient patients, immunogenic material is still detected. Two proteins, X and Y, are clearly seen indicating the presence of C-II-like proteins. Similarly, the presence of C-II reactivity in the C-II-Padova probands was detected by immunoblotting [35].

An answer to the question of the significance of C-II iummunoreactivity in the original Canadian carriers has recently been proposed. Connelly and coworkers [8] have been able to describe the full sequence of the mutant Apo C-II named *Apo C-II-Toronto*. It is a 74-amino-acid version of Apo C-II. Due to a frame-shift mutation, the code for Apo C-II leads to a stop-codon in position 75 (Fig. 3). This is most likely a deletional mutant caused by the loss of one single base, either a guanine or a thymine, in the preceding codon resulting in the stop-codon at position 75 and introducing a cysteine in position 74. The question remains why the C-II-Toronto is nonfunctional. Since the serine protease activity of Apo C-II, located in the 55–67 amino acid stretch, is normal in this mutant, it is possible that the carboxy terminal of the mutant molecule is more lipophilic than that of the corresponding portion of normal C-II, thus leading to some kind of distorted interaction between the Apo C-II-Toronto and lipids. Recently, Connelly at al. have also been able to describe another Canadian mutant, the Apo C-II-St. Michael, associated with both hypertriglyceridemia and arterial disease, a new finding among C-II-deficient cases. In this case too (P.W. Connelly, personal communication) the emergency of a stop-codon is the final mechanism. As yet there is no full information on the Apo C-II-Padova, although here also there is evidence of a posttranslational defect with production of a molecule of reduced size [35].

In conclusion, we have at least three or four mutants of Apo C-II, all of which are associated with hypertriglyceridemia and only one of which (the Apo C-II-St. Michael) is associated with arterial disease. All seem to exhibit some sort of abnormality in the protein. For the present, however, we can conclude that there is no clearcut Apo C-Il deficiency, but that some significant hypertriglyceridemic syndromes are related to abnormalities in the C-II protein.

69   74   76

C-II

Asp Gln Val Leu Ser Val Leu Lys
GAC CAA GTT CTT TCT GTG CTG AAG

C-II Toronto

Thr Lys Phe Phe Leu Cys
ACC AAG TTC TTT CTG TGC   TGA

Fig. 3. Genomic and amino acid sequence of normal C-II and Apo C-II Toronto in the 69–76 amino acid stretch. Probably because of a base deletion, a one base shift occurs in the C-II Toronto mutant, leading to a stop codon (TGA) after amino acid 74 [8]

HDL Deficiencies

HDL are an ideal tool for the study of deficiencies or mutations. In the case of HDL, in fact, we have acquired the most information in terms of the biological significance of lipoprotein particles. The association of one kind of HDL particle or another with arterial disease and/or protection from arterial disease is well known. It is interesting to note that in several syndromes associated with Apo A-I mutants, small HDL are present, linked to apparent good health and even cardiovascular protection.

HDL deficiency may, in many cases, be a *secondary syndrome*, i.e. linked to hypertriglyceridemia, nicotine abuse, physical inactivity, etc. The *primary deficiencies* are also numerous: Tangier disease, fish-eye disease, A-I-C-III deficiencies (variants I and II), some of the mutants, and HDL processing defects.

Tangier disease is not related to a mutant apolipoprotein but has important clinical consequences, widely known to investigators in this field [12]. Tangier disease is characterized by diffuse cholesteryl ester deposition, hepatosplenomegaly, peripheral neuropathy, and corneal opacifications. The major biochemical abnormalities are a virtually complete absence of normal HDL and marked reduction of Apo A-I in plasma [29]. The DNA sequence of the Apo A-I gene shows no clear alterations in these patients, possibly only with the single base substitution (G→T), resulting in the isosteric replacement of a glutamic acid residue at position 120 with aspartic acid [28].

Among the early theories on the mechanism of development of Tangier disease was that of a defect in the processing of pro-Apo A-I. This undergoes complex intra- and extracellular processing, and pro-Apo A-I is usually present in small amounts in plasma. Evidence indicated that pro-Apo A-I was abnormally processed in Tangier plasma [32]. This hypothesis, however, was later not confirmed, and processing of pro-Apo A-I is now believed to be normal. Recent hypotheses underline a potential defect in the macrophage processing of HDL. Actually I must say that I was probably the first to suggest, as a joke, that macrophages might be sick in Tangier patients. The Münster group has clearly shown that macrophages have the capacity to interact with HDL as well as with acetyl-LDL [33]. In contrast, however, to LDL, which wind up in lysosomes, HDL are interiorized by a variety of membranous particles, thus leading to recycling and eventual elimination of HDL. This hypothesis leads to postulating the existence of a so-called HDL receptor. Although I personally fail to see the physiological necessity for an HDL receptor, there are still a variety of contributions indicating that there may be some protein with molecular weight x of around 110 kd capable of binding HDL [23]. Possibly, the molecular defect of Tangier disease lies in this complex extra- and intracellular pathway [34], but there are conflicting views. Recently the unusual A-II richness of VLDL in Tangier patients was underlined [37]. Tangier disease may just be a heterogeneous disorder and there may be different errors in different individuals.

Fish-eye disease (FED) was detected in a Swedish kindred. Severe corneal opacification and a marked reduction of HDL and Apo A-I are its major features [5]. Studies on the genome have failed to detect any significant alterations [27]. FED, similarly to the A-I-Milano mutant, is characterized by the presence of very small HDL particles. By gradient gel electrophoresis, subjects with FED show HDL of 3b–3c mobility, vs

2b–3a in most normals [5]. Individuals with FED, again, similarly to the A-I-Milano carriers, have no significant arterial disease.

One interesting property of FED plasma is its poor capacity to activate cholesterol esterification [6]. Specifically it will not activate the formation of cholesterol esters in HDL, but it will do so in other lipoproteins. FED plasma lacks, therefore, α-HDL lecithin: cholesterol acyltransferase (LCAT), although β-LCAT is present in normal amounts.

Among the HDL deficiency syndromes, the one most clearly associated with arterial disease is the so-called *A-I-C-III deficiency*. This syndrome is characterized by early and severe coronary atherosclerosis with tendon and cutaneous xanthomata and corneal opacities [25]. Biochemically, the first two carriers, two young sisters, had normal total plasma cholesterol and triglyceride, but dramatically reduced HDL-cholesterol (4 and 7 mg/dl) and only traces of Apo A-I and Apo C-III in plasma. Southern blotting of the genomic cDNA from the probands, after Eco RI digestion and hybridization with an Apo A-I cDNA probe, revealed a single 6.5-kb band, instead of the 13-kb band in normals [16]. Relatives showed both the 6.5- and the 13-kb bands, thus suggesting homozygosity in the two sisters and heterozygosity in the other family members. The genomic abnormality is not the consequence of single base pair substitutions, but rather of a more extensive DNA alteration. The complex rearrangement of the A-I-C-III gene in these patients has been recently characterized [17].

Another similar syndrome, initially named *"Apo A-I absence,"* was detected in a 45-year-old woman with severe angina who died after coronary bypass surgery. At autopsy, significant atherosclerosis in the coronary and pulmonary arteries and in the abdominal aorta, as well as stromal lipid depositions in the cornea, were detected [30]. Genomic analysis failed to show any significant alterations. It has been proposed that these two phenotypically similar syndromes, be named familial apolipoprotein A-I and C-III deficiencies, variants I and II [30]. However, Ordovas (personal communication) recently suggested that apolipoprotein A-I-C-III deficiency variant II is due to a large deletion in the A-I-C-III gene cluster which results in mild abnormalities in the heterozygotes but in a severe deficiency in the homozygotes. The reason for the difficulty in establishing the cause of this alteration was the early death of the homozygous carrier.

Going finally to the *A-I mutations,* we find a long list of abnormalities, most coming from the Federal Republic of Germany, one from Italy, and one from Norway, this being the only homozygous case [20]. In most of these there is no obvious biochemical abnormality, except for the *A-I-Milano* which is characterized by a significant reduction of HDL-cholesterol levels. This mutant, first identified in a 47-year-old Italian man [9] has a cysteine for arginine replacement at position 173 of Apo A-I. The A-I-Milano may be present in the form of monomers, dimers ($A-I_M-A-I_M$), or complexes with Apo A-II ($A-I_M-A-II$) [37]. Up to now a total of 33 carriers, ranging in age from 5 to 85 years, have been identified, all descending from a single mating couple living at the end of the eighteenth century [14]. All carriers are heterozygotes, and the variant is transmitted as an autosomal codominant trait. Multiple biochemical abnormalities are detected: markedly reduced levels of HDL-cholesterol (between 7–33 mg/dl), as well as of Apo A-I and Apo A-II; hypertriglyceridemia; triglyceride enrichment of LDL and HDL; nearly total absence of the HDL_2 subfraction, with anomalous, dense, polydisperse HDL_3 [10].

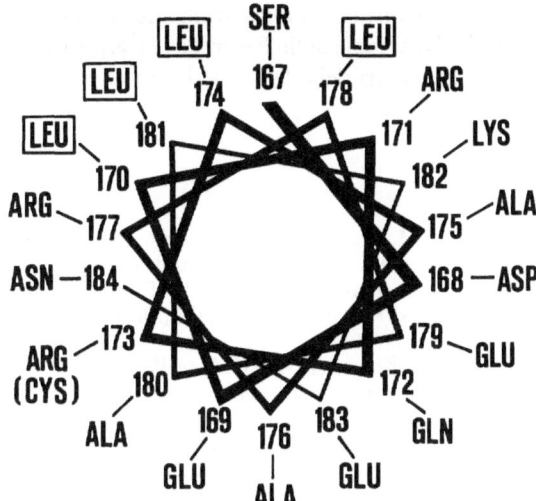

Fig. 4. Helical wheel presentation of the presumed structure of segment 167–184 of apolipoprotein A-I. In the Apo A-I-Milano mutant, Arg[173] is substituted with cysteine. This substitution leads to the disappearance of an ion pair, Glu[169]-Arg[173], with a resulting loss in amphipathic structure and lipid binding capacity [11]

Since, in spite of the numerous biochemical risk factors for vascular disease (low HDL, Apo A-I, A-I/B ratio, etc), no significant vascular pathologies are present in the carriers, several studies have been performed to investigate the behavior of the abnormal A-I-Milano. Results of structural studies are compatible with a reduced number of helical segments involved in lipid association (Fig. 4). These data suggest that the mutant protein might have more efficient uptake capacities for tissue lipids, thus explaining the relative protection against vascular disease despite the presence of very low HDL levels [11].

Recently, in vitro studies have shown that the A-I-Milano carriers have a remarkably stable HDL system. In fact, the small HDL$_3$, prevalent in these subjects, are modified to a very limited extent following exposure to triglyceride-rich particles. Other studies concerning the possible presence of specific restriction fragment length polymorphisms have, as yet, failed to disclose any specific abnormality.

Conclusion

Lipoprotein deficiency syndromes provide clinicians and investigators in the lipoprotein field with a remarkable model for the study of lipoprotein function and of the impact of genetic factors on lipoprotein metabolism. A gross evaluation of these abnormalities suggest that in most cases there is no evidence of significant clinical consequences; less than half of these syndromes are associated with some form, occasionally severe, of arterial disease. The A-I-Milano mutant seems to be associated with some protection from atherosclerosis. Further studies are necessary to detect specific associations of these abnormalities with more general alterations in the genome, thus possibly explaining the evolutionary significance of apolipoprotein mutants.

Acknowledgements. Studies from the author's laboratory were supported by the Consiglio Nazionale delle Ricerche of Italy, Progetto Finalizzato Ingegneria Genetica e Basi Molecolari delle Malattie Ereditarie.

References

1. Anchors JM, Gregg RE, Law SW, Brewer HB Jr (1986) Apo E deficiency: markedly decreased levels of cellular Apo E mRNA. Biochem Biophys Res Commun 134: 937–943
2. Baggio G, Manzato E, Gabellic, Fellin R, Martini S, Baldi E, Verlato F, Baiocchi MR, Sprecher DL, Kashyap ML, Brewer HB Jr, Crepaldi G (1986) Apolipoprotein C-II deficiency syndrome. J Clin Invest 77: 520–527
3. Bassen FA, Kornzweig AL (1950) Malformation of the erythrocytes in a case of atypical retinitis pigmentosa. Blood 5: 381–387
4. Breckenridge WC, Little JA, Steiner G, Chow A, Poast M (1978) Hypertriglyceridemia associated with deficiency of apolipoprotein C-II. N Engl J Med 298: 1265–1273
5. Carlson LA (1982) Fish eye disease: a new familial condition with massive corneal opacities and dyslipoproteinemia. Eur J Clin Invest 12: 41–53
6. Carlson LA, Holmquist L (1985) Evidence for deficiency of high-density lipoprotein lecithin-cholesterol acyltransferase activity (α-LCAT) in Fish Eye disease. Acta Med Scand 218: 189–196
7. Cladaras C, Hadzopoulou-Cladaras M, Felber BK, Powlakis G, Zannis VI (1987) The molecular basis of a familial Apo E deficiency. J Biol Chem 262: 2310–2315
8. Connelly PW, Maguire GF, Hofmann T, Little JA (1987) Structure of apolipoprotein C-II-Toronto a nonfunctional human apolipoprotein. Proc Natl Acad Sci USA 84: 270–273
9. Franceschini G, Sirtori CR, Capurso A, Weisgraber KH, Mahley RW (1980) Apoprotein A-I-Milano: decreased high density lipoprotein cholesterol with significant lipoprotein modifications and without clinical atherosclerosis in an Italian family. J Clin Invest 66: 892–900
10. Franceschini G, Frosi TG, Manzoni C, Gianfranceschi G, Sirtori CR (1982) High density lipoprotein-3 heterogeneity in subjects with the Apo A-I-Milano variant. J Biol Chem 257: 9926–9930
11. Franceschini G, Vecchio G, Gianfranceschi G, Magani G, Sirtori CR (1985) Apolipoprotein A-I-Milano. Accelerated binding and dissociation from lipids of a human apolipoprotein variant. J Biol Chem 260: 16321–16325
12. Fredrickson DS (1965) The inheritance of high density lipoprotein deficiency (Tangier disease). J Clin Invest 44: 228–237
13. Ghiselli GC, Schaefer EJ, Gascon P, Brewer HB Jr (1981) Type III hyperlipoproteinemia associated with plasma apolipoprotein E deficiency. Science 214: 1239–1241
14. Gualandri V, Franceschini G, Sirtori CR, Gianfranceschi G, Orsini GB, Cerrone A, Menotti A (1985) A-I Milano apoprotein. Identification of the complete kindred and evidence of a dominant genetic transmission. Am J Hum Genet 37: 1083–1097
15. Hospattankar AV, Fairwell T, Ronan R, Brewer HB Jr (1983) Amino acid sequences of human apolipoprotein C-II from normal and hyperlipoproteinemic subjects. J Biol Chem 259: 318–322
16. Karathanasis SK, Norum RA, Zannis VI, Breslow JL (1983) An inherited polymorphism in the human apolipoprotein A-I gene locus related to the development of atherosclerosis. Nature 301: 718–720
17. Karathanasis SK, Ferris E, Haddad I (1987) DNA inversion within the apolipoproteins A-I/C-III/A-IV-encoding gene cluster of certain patients with premature atherosclerosis. Proc Natl Acad Sci USA 84: 7198–7202
18. Lackner KJ, Monge JC, Gregg RE, Hoeg JM, Triche TJ, Law SW, Brewer HB Jr (1986) Analysis of the apolipoprotein B gene and messenger ribonucleic acid in abetalipoproteinemia. J Clin Invest 78: 1707–1712
19. Maguire GF, Little JA, Kakis G, Breckenridge WC (1984) Apolipoprotein C-II deficiency associated with nonfunctional mutant forms of apolipoprotein C-II. Can J Biochem 62: 847–852
20. Mahley RW, Innerarity TL, Rall SC Jr, Weisgraber KH (1984) Plasma lipoproteins: apolipoprotein structure and function. J Lipid Res 25: 1277–1294

21. Malloy MJ, Kane JP, Hardman DA, Hamilton RL, Dalal KB (1981) Normotriglyceridemic abetalipoproteinemia. Absence of the B-100 apolipoprotein. J Clin Invest 67: 1441–1450
22. Malloy MJ, Kane JP (1982) Hypolipidemia. Med Clin North Am 66: 469–484
23. Monaco L, Bond HM, Howell KE, Cortese RL (1987) A recombinant Apo A-I-protein. A hybrid reproduces the binding of HDL to its receptor. EMBO J 6: 3253–3260
24. Müller DPR, Lloyd JK (1982) Effects of large oral doses of vitamin E on the neurological sequelae of patients with abetalipoproteinemia. Ann NY Acad Sci 393: 133–144
25. Norum RA, Lakier JB, Goldstein S, Angel A, Goldberg RB, Block WD, Noffze DK, Dolphin PJ, Edelglass J, Bogorad DD, Alaupovic P (1982) Familial deficiency of apolipoprotein A-I and C-II and precocious coronary-artery disease. N Engl J Med 306: 1513–1519
26. Rall SC Jr, Weisgraber KH, Innerarity TL, Mahley RW (1982) Structural basis for receptor binding heterogeneity of apolipoprotein E from type III hyperlipoproteinemic subjects. Proc Natl Acad Sci USA 79: 4696–4700
27. Rees A, Stocks J, Shoulders C, Carlson LA, Baralle FE, Galton DJ (1984) Restriction enzyme analysis of the apolipoprotein A-I gene in Fish Eye Disease and Tangier Disease. Acta Med Scand 215: 235–237
28. Rees A, Stocks J, Sharpe CR, Vella MA, Shoulders CC, Katz J, Jowett NI, Baralle FE, Galton DJ (1985) Deoxyribonucleic acid polymorphisms in the apolipoprotein A-I-C-III gene cluster. J Clin Invest 76: 1090–1095
29. Schaefer EJ (1984) The clinical, biochemical and genetic features in familial disorders of high density lipoprotein deficiency. Arteriosclerosis 4: 302–322
30. Schaefer EJ, Ordovas EM, Law SW, Ghiselli GC, Kashyap MT, Srivastava LS, Heaton WH, Albers JJ, Connor WE, Lindgren FT, Lemeshev Y, Segrest JP, Brewer HB Jr (1985) Familial apolipoprotein A-I and C-III deficiency, variant II. J Lipid Res 26: 1089–1101
31. Schaefer ES, Gregg RE, Ghiselli GC, Forte TM, Ordovas JM, Zech LA, Brewer HB Jr (1986) Familial apolipoprotein E deficiency. J Clin Invest 78: 1206–1219
32. Schmitz G, Assmann G, Rall SC Jr, Mahley RW (1983) Tangier disease: defective recombination of a specific Tangier apolipoprotein AI-isoform (pro-Apo A-I) with high density lipoproteins. Proc Natl Acad Sci USA 80: 6081–6085
33. Schmitz G, Robeneck H, Lohmann V, Assmann G (1985) Interactions of high-density lipoproteins with cholesteryl ester-laden macrophages: biochemical and morphological characterization of cell surface receptor binding, endocytosis and resecretion of high density lipoproteins by macrophages. EMBO J 4: 613–622
34. Schmitz G, Assmann G, Robenek H, Brennhausen B (1985) Tangier disease: a disorder of intracellular membrane traffic. Proc Natl Acad Sci USA 82: 6305–6309
35. Sprecher DL, Taam L, Brewer HB Jr (1984) Two dimensional electrophoresis of human plasma apolipoproteins. Clin Chem 30: 2084–2092
36. Steinberg DS, Grundy SM, Mok AYI, Turner JD, Weinstein DB, Albers JJ (1979) Metabolic studies in an unusual case of asymptomatic familial hypobetalipoproteinemia with hypoalphalipoproteinemia and fasting chylomicronemia. J Clin Invest 64: 292–301
37. Wang C-S, Alaupovic P, Gregg RE, Brewer HB Jr (1987) Studies on the mechanism of hypertriglyceridemia in Tangier disease. Determination of plasma lipolytic activities, K_1 values and apolipoprotein composition of the major lipoprotein density classes. Biochem Biophys Acta 920: 9–19
38. Weisgraber KH, Rall SC Jr, Bersot TP, Mahley RW, Franceschini G, Sirtori CR (1983) Apolipoprotein A-I-Milano: detection of normal A-I in affected subjects and evidence for a cysteine for arginine substitution in the variant A-I. J Biol Chem 258: 2808–2513
39. Young SG, Bertics SJ, Curtiss LK, Witztum JL (1987) Characterization of an abnormal species of apolipoprotein B, apolipoprotein B-37, associated with familial hypobetalipoproteinemia. J Clin Invest 79: 1831–1841
40. Young SG, Bertics SJ, Curtiss LK, Dubois BW, Witztum JL (1987) Genetic analysis of a kindred with familial hypobetalipoproteinemia. J Clin Invest 79: 1842–1851

Significance of the Interaction Between Lipoprotein Subfractions and Macrophages for Reverse Cholesterol Transport

G. Schmitz, and H. Robenek

Plasma high-density lipoproteins (HDL) represent a highly heterogeneous group of particles which are involved in a number of metabolic processes including steroidogenesis, bile salt formation, cholesterol uptake, the binding of cholesterol ester transfer protein (CETP), and reverse cholesterol transport. The precursors of plasma HDL originate from the intestine or the liver, and upon formation of HDL_3 particles, tissue cholesterol is generated and included into the particles.

It has been hypothesized that HDL absorb unesterified cholesterol by physicochemical mechanisms from macrophage cell membranes and other cholesterol-enriched cells. This leads to an imbalance between cytoplasmic cholesterol and cell surface cholesterol; equilibrium is restored by movement of cholesterol from the cytoplasmic pool.

In addition, cholesterol accumulation in macrophages, mediated by modified lipoproteins (e. g., acetylated low-density lipoprotein, AcLDL), stimulates these cells to synthesize and secrete apolipoprotein (Apo) E/phospholipid discs. During the intraplasmatic cholesterol esterification process mediated by lecithin:cholesterol acyltransferase (LCAT), HDL are assumed to incorporate unesterified cholesterol from the cell surface and Apo E from secreted Apo E/phospholipid discs and thereby mediate reverse cholesterol transport from peripheral cells back to the liver. The resulting cholesteryl ester- and Apo E-enriched HDL_1 are transported to the liver where they may be recognized by a hepatic Apo E receptor.

In collaboration with Dr. Robenek we have made a detailed study of the mechanism of cholesterol transfer from macrophages to HDL particles using biochemical and morphological methods. We demonstrated that in addition to a physicochemical exchange of cholesterol from the cells to HDL_3, there is a high-affinity binding site for Apo A-I-containing HDL which shows saturation kinetics (Fig. 1). The Scatchard plot of the binding curve indicates a single class of binding sites. HDL which bind to this high-affinity binding site are internalized into nonlysosomal organelles (Fig. 1). Evidence for the internalization of the HDL particles results in part from electron-microscopic experiments with gold-labeled HDL which allow the intracellular route of the HDL particles to be followed. Additional evidence for HDL internalization comes from anti-Apo A-I immunoperoxidase staining of thin sections from macrophages previously exposed to nonlabeled HDL and from fluorescence-labeled HDL_3 (RITC-HDL_3), quantitated by flow cytometry or analyzed by fluorescence microscopy at 4°C and 37°C.

As a result of our studies we hypothesize that acetylated LDL and HDL follow different pathways in the macrophage (Fig. 2):

H. U. Klör (Ed.)
Lipoprotein Subfractions
Omega-3 Fatty Acids
© Springer-Verlag Berlin Heidelberg 1989

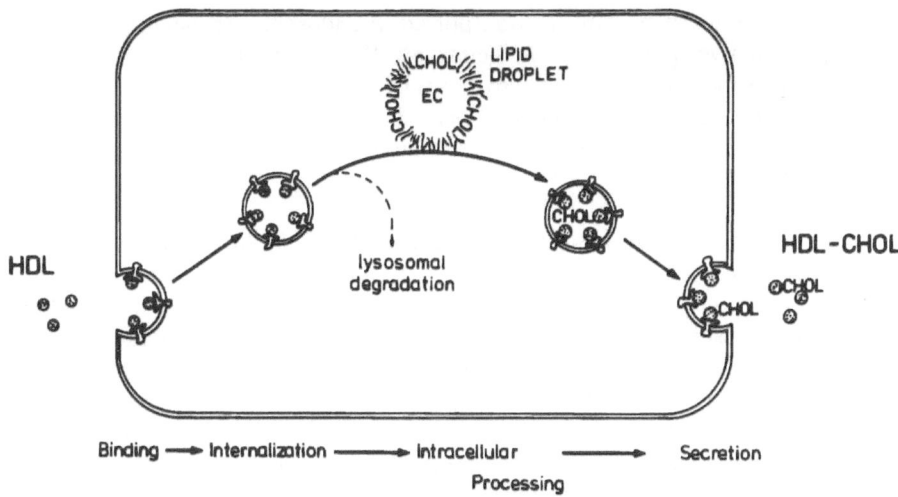

Fig. 1. Interaction of HDL with macrophages. *EC = esterified cholesterol*

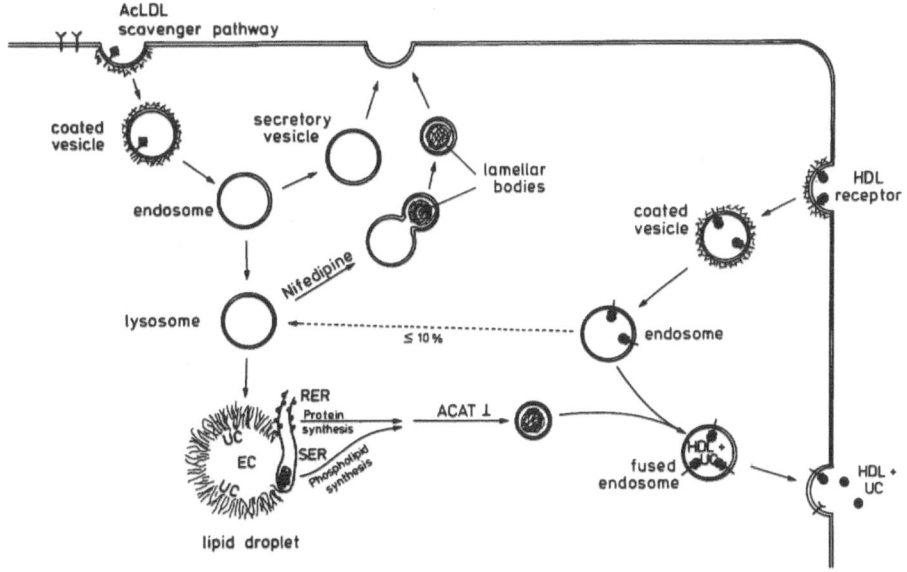

Fig. 2. Cholesterol metabolism in macrophages. *AcLDL,* Acetyl LDL; *EC = esterified cholesterol; UC = unesterified cholesterol; RER, SER,* rough, smooth endoplasmic reticulum

- Acetylated LDL bind to the scavenger receptor, are internalized via coated pits and coated vesicles, and are directed to lysosomes where the whole particle is degraded. The cholesterol moiety is transported to the cytoplasm and may be stored in the form of cytoplasmic lipid droplets or released from the cell.
- HDL$_3$ bind to specific binding sites and are internalized via coated pits and coated vesicles. However, in contrast to acetylated LDL, HDL are not significantly

degraded in lysosomes, but are transported in endosomes through the cell and secreted as native lipoproteins. On their transcellular route HDL come into contact with cytoplasmic lipid droplets where they take up cholesterol and Apo E, and they are secreted as cholesterol- and Apo E-rich HDL. This pathway can be amplified by stimulation of protein kinase C or by inhibition of the cholesterol-esterifying enzyme ACAT.

The interaction of HDL with the lipid droplets has been further investigated by morphological methods (Fig. 3). Upon lipid accumulation in the macrophage, an intimate contact between the endoplasmic reticulum (ER) and the margin of the lipid droplet can be observed. At the site of contact, due to the induction of phospholipid and apolipoprotein synthesis, "lamellar bodies" are formed which are surrounded by a newly synthesized membrane. These lamellar bodies consist of free cholesterol, phospholipids, and apolipoproteins including Apo E. From these lamellar bodies, HDL take up cholesterol, Apo E, and phospholipids on their route through the cell (Fig. 3b). In the absence of HDL, the lamellar bodies which originate from cytoplasmic lipid droplets, cannot be secreted from the cell.

We could isolate two HDL-binding proteins: a 78-kDa protein from human placenta and a 110-kDa HDL-binding protein from human leukocytes. Investigations concerning the ligand specificity of the 110-kDa protein revealed that the affinity for

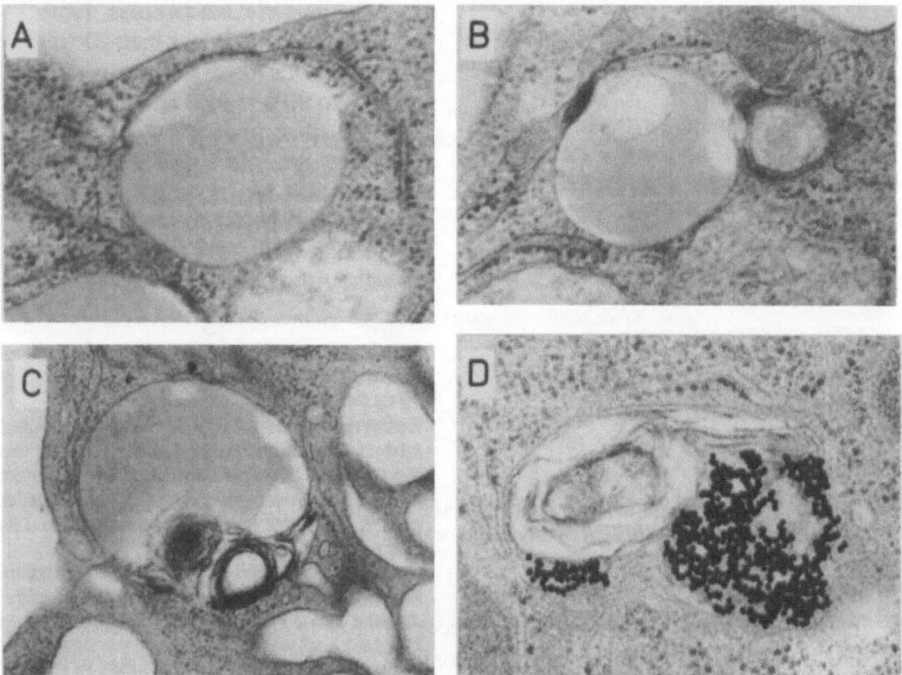

Fig. 3A–D. Cholesterol release from lipid droplets in macrophages: At the margin of lipid droplets, an intimate contact with endoplasmatic reticulum can be observed **(A)**. At the site of contact, "lamellar bodies" are formed **(B, C)**. Gold-labelled HDL are in close contact to these lamellar bodies **(D)**

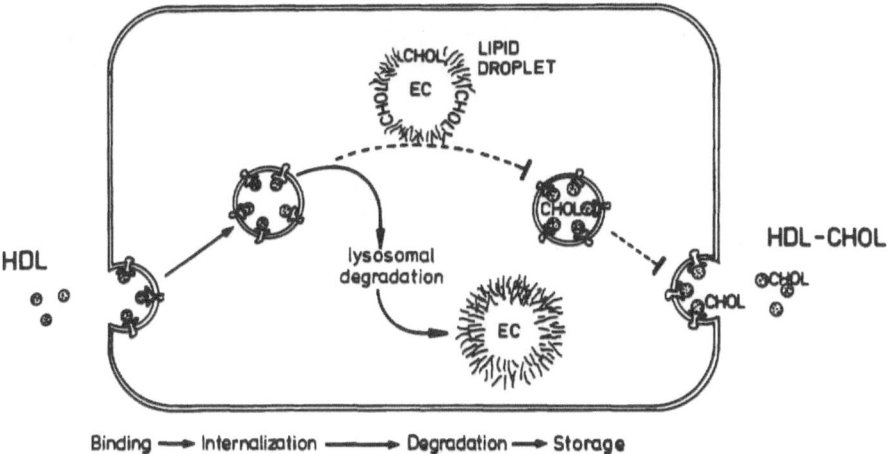

Fig. 4. HDL pathway in Tangier macrophages. *EC = esterified cholesterol*

discoidal HDL precursors is higher than that for the spherical Apo A-I-containing HDL particles. From analysis of the HDL binding sites on human leukocytes by fluorescence flow cytometry using RITC-HDL, we found that granulocytes show the highest HDL binding, followed by monocytes, while lymphocytes have a lower HDL receptor activity.

In Tangier disease, a rare disorder with complete lack of HDL in the plasma associated with splenomegaly, enlarged tonsils, and lipid storage in the cells of the reticuloendothelial system but no elevated risk for atherosclerosis, the disturbances of cellular cholesterol homeostasis were studied in detail. In patients with Tangier disease there is a normal rate of Apo A-I synthesis, a normal primary structure of Apo A-I, normal conversion from pro-Apo A-I to mature Apo A-I, and normal association of Tangier Apo A-I with normal HDL, while HDL are completely absent and there is a decreased Apo A-I concentration (< 2% of normal). In these patients accelerated catabolism of HDL has been postulated. Our own experiments showed that Tangier patients may suffer from a disorder of intracellular transport of HDL or its precursors (Fig. 4).

Binding of normal HDL to Tangier monocyte/macrophages is higher than in controls, and HDL are erroneously directed to lysosomal degradation, leading to lipid storage in the cytoplasmic compartment. This leads to diminished release of cholesterol from lipid droplets by the HDL receptor-dependent mechanism. In these patients we detected another HDL-independent cholesterol release from lipid-loaded macrophages (Fig. 5).

Upon cholesterol influx lysosomal foamy organelles are transformed into lamellar bodies, and the whole lysosome is transformed into small vesicles with a grapelike structure. These lamellar bodies can be directly secreted from the cell, have a diameter of 200–300 Å, and are rich in free cholesterol and phospholipids (68% free cholesterol, 21% phospholipids, three-fourths of which is PC (phosphatidylcholine),

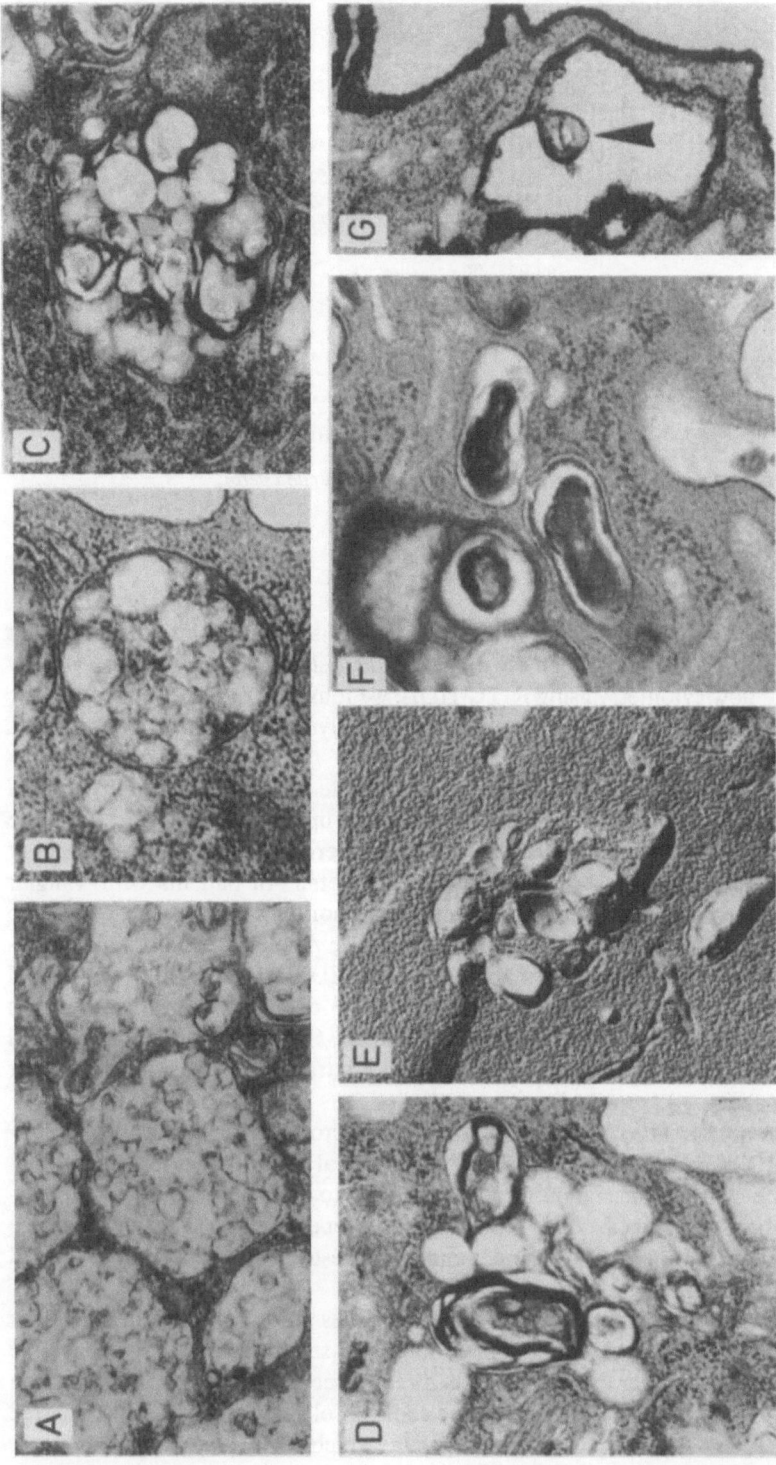

Fig. 5A–G. Cholesterol release from lysosomes in macrophages. Upon cholesterol accumulation, foamy organelles originating from lysosomes are transformed into "lamellar bodies" (A–D) revealing a grape-like structure (E, freeze fracture). These lamellar bodies are actively secreted from the cells (F, G)

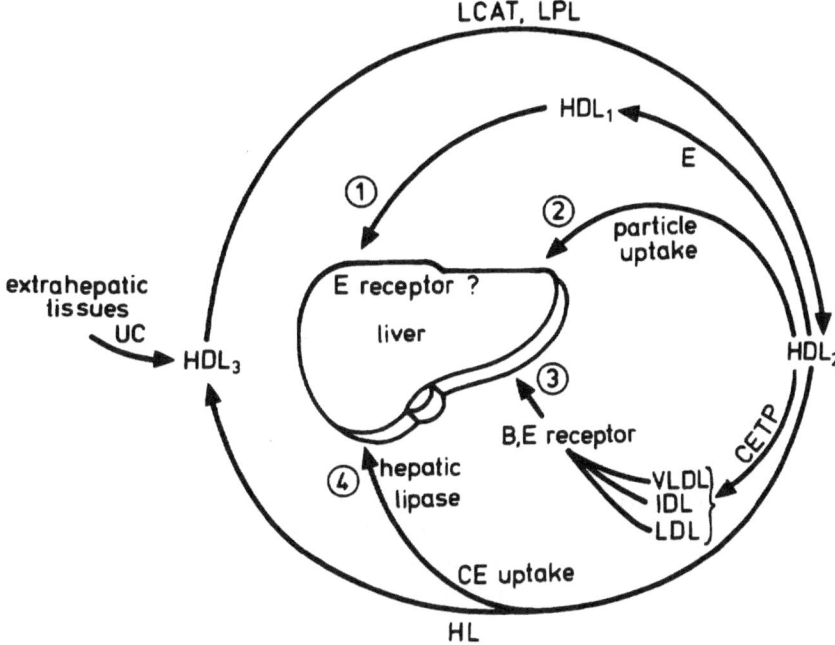

Fig. 6. Major pathways of reverse cholesterol transport. *CE = esterified cholesterol;* *HL,* hepatic lipase; *UC,* unesterified cholesterol

one fourth SPM (sphingomyelin). This HDL-independent release of cholesterol can be amplified by stimulation of protein kinase A or by calcium antagonists (e. g., nifedipine).

Both the HDL-dependent and the HDL-independent pathway protect the macrophage and maybe other cholesterol-loaded cells from overaccumulation of cholesterol and foam cell formation. Cholesterol accumulation and inflammatory activation trigger the macrophage to synthesize and secrete a large variety of secretory products including enzymes, proteins, and growth factors for fibroblasts, endothelial cells, and smooth muscle cells which enhance the atherosclerotic process.

The cholesterol-enriched HDL secreted by the cells initially enter the HDL_3 fraction of the plasma compartment, where they are metabolized by the action of LCAT and lipoprotein lipase to HDL_2. In the first of the four major pathways postulated for reverse cholesterol transport to the liver (Fig. 6), HDL_2 are further converted to HDL_1 which may be taken up by the postulated hepatic E receptor. The second pathway may involve a receptor-mediated mechanism which recognizes Apo A-I-containing HDL taken up by the liver. The third pathway acts via CETP, which is transferred from HDL particles to Apo B-containing lipoproteins and thereby leads cholesterol into the B, E receptor route. The fourth pathway may involve hepatic lipase which interacts with HDL particles and mediates a selective uptake of cholesteryl ester into the liver.

HDL Receptor of Cultured Adipocytes and Its Role in Reverse Cholesterol Transport

G. AILHAUD

It is known that among peripheral tissues adipose tissue is able to store a large pool of unesterified cholesterol and, when needed, to mobilize it. As previously shown by A. Angel and colleagues, approximately 40% of the total body cholesterol is located in adipose tissue in normal man. This figure can be as high as 65%–70% in the obese state.

In rodents taken as animal models, the cholesterol pool of adipose tissue is present in unesterified form and localized to the bulk triglyceride storage droplets. The cholesterol content increases with age, diet, and state of obesity.

There is a six- to sixty-fold higher cholesterol content, expressed in mg/g of protein, in the adipose tissue than in any other organ. This pool of cholesterol can be mobilized quite rapidly and to a large extent during starvation, which implies that some kind of reverse cholesterol transport should take place *in vivo*. The fact that adipose tissue is able to store and mobilize a large pool of cholesterol indicates that the control of cholesterol homeostatis in this tissue is very loose indeed.

In order to study reverse cholesterol transport at the cellular level, since adipocytes show a viability limited to a few hours *in vitro*, we have established in our laboratory preadipocyte cell lines from genetically obese mice (Ob17 line and subclones) and their lean counterparts (HGFu line). First, the cells of these established lines are able to differentiate *in vitro* into adipose cells with morphological and biochemical characteristics of rodent adipocytes. Second, these cells are able to differentiate *in vivo* when they are injected in the undifferentiated state into athymic mice. *In vitro*, as shown in Fig. 1A, fat cells are present as clusters, which can be stained for triglycerides at the cellular level with Oil-Red-O. *In vivo*, a few weeks after injection, the cells develop into a fat pad, and mature adipocytes can be easily seen on semi-thin sections of the fat pad (Fig. 1B).

We have studied the binding parameters of lipoprotein receptor sites in mouse Ob17 adipose cells. A "classical" Apo B, E receptor is present: the binding of labeled low-density lipoprotein (LDL) is competitively inhibited by human LDL as well as mouse LDL. Methylated LDL and Apo E-free high-density lipoprotein (HDL) are not competitors. These receptor sites are present both in nondifferentiated and differentiated cells.

In differentiated Ob17 cells there is no significant cholesterol synthesis and esterification and, more importantly, no down-regulation of the Apo B, E receptor sites occurs in the presence of LDL. At the same time, the cells remain able to bind, internalize, and degrade LDL. Therefore, this lack of stringent cholesterol homeostasis should, in the presence of LDL cholesterol, lead to cholesterol accumulation. If one looks at the Apo A-I, A-II receptor sites in the same cells, the binding of labeled

H. U. Klör (Ed.)
Lipoprotein Subfractions
Omega-3 Fatty Acids
© Springer-Verlag Berlin Heidelberg 1989

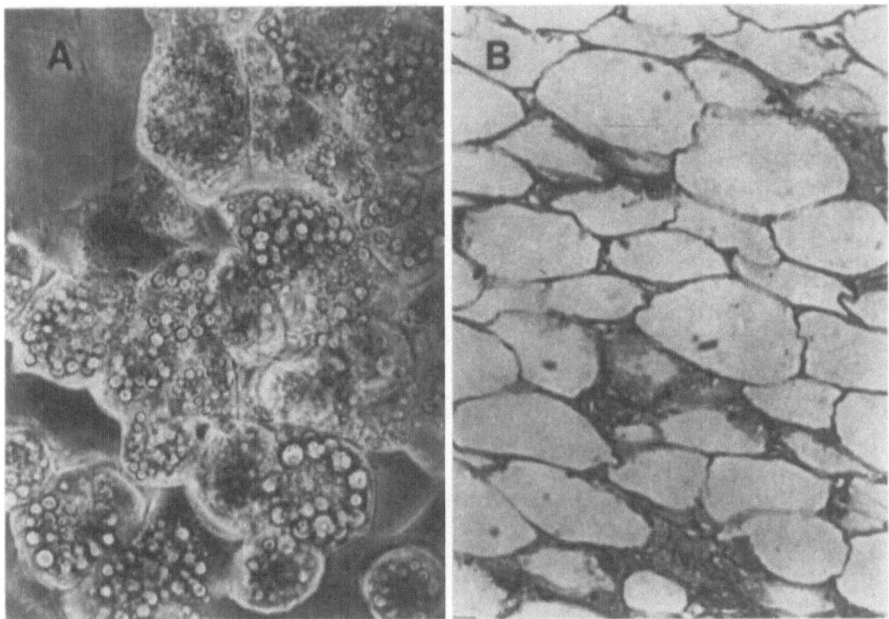

Fig. 1A, B. Clusters of fat cells stained for triglycerides at the cellular level with Oil-Red-O

Apo E-free HDL is competitively inhibited by the same unlabeled lipoprotein particles but not by LDL. The binding of labeled HDL_3 is competitively inhibited by Apo A-I proteoliposomes, mouse HDL, and unlabeled HDL_3. The binding of labeled Apo A-I or Apo A-II proteoliposomes is competitively inhibited by the unlabeled corresponding proteoliposomes; cross-competition between both proteoliposomes does also take place. Dimyristoylphosphatidylcholine (DMPC) liposomes are not competitors. As for LDL receptor sites, these receptor sites are present both in nondifferentiated and differentiated cells.

Once more it is important to note that, in differentiated cells, there is no upregulation of the Apo A-I, A-II receptor sites in the presence of LDL, whereas HDL, in contrast to LDL, are not degraded.

In conclusion, there is again a lack of stringent cholesterol homeostasis, and therefore, providing that the cells are preloaded with cholesterol, a mobilization of cholesterol should take place.

Both predictions of cholesterol accumulation and mobilization are fulfilled. If one considers the kinetics of cholesterol accumulation in differentiated Ob1771 cells, the accumulation occurs only in the presence of LDL, as expected. There is a very fast cholesterol efflux from cholesterol preloaded cells in the presence of HDL_3 or Apo A-I proteoliposomes. In the absence of Apo A-I proteoliposomes, there is no efflux whatsoever (Fig. 2). As a matter of fact, the rate of cholesterol efflux in these cells is many times higher than that reported for other cell types (fibroblasts, endothelial cells). Dose-response curves for cholesterol accumulation (via LDL) and cholesterol mobilization (via HDL_3 or Apo A-I) show that the half-maximally effective concen-

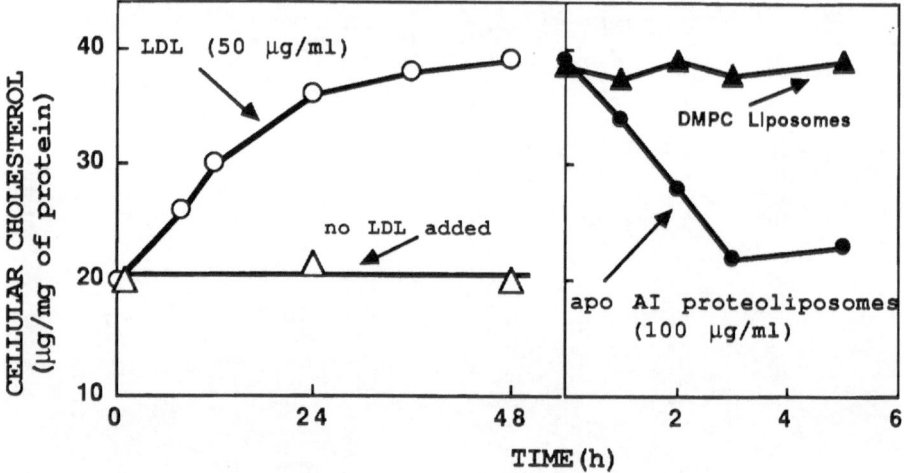

Fig. 2. Cholesterol accumulation in differentiated Ob 1771 cells

trations are in good agreement with the apparent K_d value of binding to their respective receptor sites, strongly suggesting the critical role of the LDL and HDL receptor sites in cholesterol accumulation and mobilization, respectively.

Apo A-I-DMPC liposomes do promote cholesterol efflux, whether or not cholesterol is included in the liposomes, whereas, in contrast, Apo A-II-DMPC liposomes, which bind also to the cell surface, do not promote any cholesterol efflux. Incidently, the presence of lecithin:cholesterol acyltransferase (LCAT) under our conditions does not seem to be required for cholesterol efflux, because similar results can be obtained in serum-free medium. Thus, these experiments tell us that Apo A-I behaves as an agonist and Apo A-II behaves as an antagonist of cholesterol efflux.

After preloading Ob1771 cells with LDL cholesterol, the cholesterol efflux was followed in the presence of LP-A-I particles or in the presence of LPA-I:A-II particles. LP-A-I particles only seem to be efficient, whatever might be the concentration of both kinds of lipoprotein particles. Control experiments show that both LP-A-I and LPA-I:A-II particles are indeed competitors of labeled HDL_3 for the binding to HDL receptor sites at the cell surface, excluding the lack of recognition of LP-A-I:A-II particles to explain their lack of effect.

What is the role of this HDL receptor in reverse cholesterol transport? It is possible to introduce genetic alterations of the growth-control mechanisms by transforming Ob1771 cells with the early region of polyomavirus. When the binding parameters of the HDL receptor sites are examined in the parental Ob17 cells and transformed Ob17PY cells, binding parameters for Apo A-I, Apo A-II, and HDL_3 can be determined in the parental line. However, no binding is detected in growing Ob17PY cells. If these cells are growth-arrested, then the maximal capacity of binding for Apo A-I, Apo A-II and HDL_3 is recovered. The lack of binding activity in intact, growing Ob17PY cells is not due to redistribution or masking of the binding sites within the cells, because crude membranes before and after solubilization do not exhibit any binding activity. This phenomenon seems to be rather specific because two other cell-surface receptors, Apo B, E and transferrin receptors, are unaffected in both parental Ob17 cells, growing Ob17PY cells, and growth-arrested Ob17PY cells. The recovery of the binding capacity is rapid ($\sim$ 16 h) and can be prevented by actinomycin D or cycloheximide, implying that some regulation takes place at a transcriptional and/or translational level.

Thus, it has become possible to study directly whether cells which are devoid of any binding capacity are capable of promoting cholesterol efflux. In contrast to parental Ob1771 cells, growing Ob17PY cells, which remain (as anticipated) able to accumulate cholesterol, become unable to mobilize cholesterol from cholesterol-preloaded cells. When growth-arrested Ob17PY cells are recovering the binding activity, they are recovering in parallel the ability to undergo cholesterol mobilization in the presence of Apo A-I or HDL_3 but not, as expected, in the presence of Apo A-II. This result strongly suggests that Apo A-I, A-II receptor sites are indeed required for reverse cholesterol transport. The purification of the A-I, A-II binding protein(s) (or receptor sites) was initiated using extracts of Ob17MT cells which are enriched in these binding sites as compared with extracts of Ob1771 cells, and using extracts of growing Ob17PY cells in parallel. The binding of HDL_3 and that of Apo A-I-proteoliposomes was performed at each step. The scheme summarizes our strategy to purify the protein (Fig. 3). After solubilization by the detergent CHAPS, immunoaffinity chromatography of the Apo A-I (or Apo A-II)/binding protein complex to anti-Apo A-I (of Apo A-II) antibodies coupled to Sepharose 4B was performed and proved to be critical for extensive purification before running HPLC. A major band and a minor one are visible by SDS-PAGE. Both bands are absent from growing Ob17PY cells. The binding protein has an apparent molecular weight of 75 kDa as determined by HPLC on a TSK-3000 column and is able to bind HDL_3, Apo A-I, and Apo A-II, but not LDL. It is inactivated by trypsin treatment and upon storage. We hope that further experiments will shed some light on the properties of this Apo A-I/Apo A-II binding material.

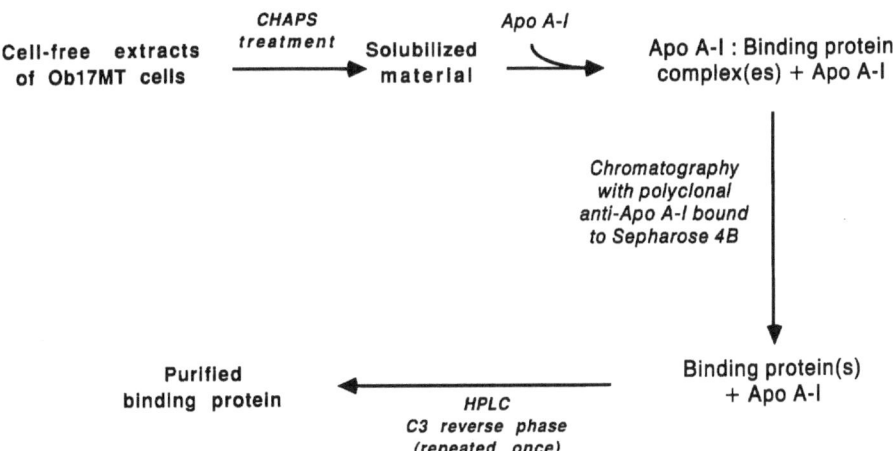

Fig. 3. Summary of strategy to purify binding protein

Omega-3 Fatty Acids

Chairmen: R. PAOLETTI, G. SCHLIERF, and H. CANZLER

Effects of Polyunsaturated Fatty Acids on Biochemical and Functional Aspects of Endothelial and Blood Cells

R. Paoletti, P. Maderna, C. Galli, and E. Tremoli

Introduction

The three major families of unsaturated fatty acids are those of oleic acid (n-9), linoleic acid (n-6) and linolenic acid (n-3). Linoleic and linolenic acid, the 18-carbon essential fatty acids obtained from the diet, are converted through desaturation and elongation steps to the long-chain polyunsaturated fatty acids (PUFAs). The 20-carbon PUFAs, dihomogammalinolenic acid (DHGLA 20:3 n-6), arachidonic acid (AA 20:4 n-6) and eicosapentaenoic acid (EPA 20:5 n-3), derived from linolenic acid, are the precursors of the prostaglandin series 1,2 and 3, respectively.

The metabolism of AA through the cyclooxygenase pathway leads to the formation of endoperoxides, unstable compounds which are transformed, in platelets, into prostaglandins, e.g. PGE_2, PGD_2, $PGF_{2\alpha}$, and into thromboxane A_2 (TXA_2) which has platelet aggregating and vasoconstrictory effects [1]. However, prostacyclin (PGI_2), the major AA metabolite formed in endothelial cells, is a potent vasodilating and antiaggregating agent [2].

EPA, the precursor of the 3 series, and, like AA, is a substrate for eicosanoid formation. In particular, EPA competitively inhibits the utilization of AA by cyclooxygenase [3]. Human platelets can convert EPA to TXA_3, which is less proaggregatory than TXA_2 [3, 4]. Additionally, EPA can be metabolized by vascular endothelium to PGI_3, which is a vasodilator and has the same platelet-inhibitory properties as PGI_2 [5].

Epidemiological Studies

Epidemiological studies revealed a lower incidence of cardiovascular disease among Greenland Eskimos than in a Scandinavian population [6, 7]. There are, in fact, some epidemiological differences in the morbidity pattern between these two populations. While stroke is probably more frequent in Eskimos than in Scandinavians, there is a very interesting reduction of acute myocardial infarction and bronchial asthma in Eskimos compared to Scandinavians [8]. This effect is related not only to genetic differences but also to diet. The Eskimo diet is poor in saturated fatty acids and rich in mono- and polyunsaturated fatty acids, with the latter dominated by n-3 PUFAs [9]. The fatty acid content of platelet phospholipids reflects the dietary intake. In fact, in platelets the level of linoleic and arachidonic acids is generally low while that of n-3 PUFAs, e.g. EPA and DHA, is several-fold higher in the Eskimo group [10]. These

H. U. Klör (Ed.)
Lipoprotein Subfractions
Omega-3 Fatty Acids
© Springer-Verlag Berlin Heidelberg 1989

changes in fatty acid content are accompanied by a reduction in triglyceride, choles-terol, low-density and very low-density lipoprotein levels and by an increase in high-density lipoprotein [9]. In addition, the elevated dietary n-3 PUFA intake results in increased levels of EPA and DHA in platelet phospholipids, with a consequent alteration in prostaglandin synthesis, accompanied by reduction of platelet aggrega-tion and by an increase in bleeding time [7, 10].

These studies suggest that a modification of diet with an increase of n-3 PUFA may be potentially important in controlling or preventing cardiovascular disease.

Effects of n-3 PUFA on Platelets and Vessel Walls

Two important events contribute to the interest in n-3 fatty acids: the epidemiological investigations carried out by Bang et al. [6] and the discovery that prostaglandins derived from EPA have biological properties different from those derived from AA [3]. Stimulated by the epidemiological findings, many investigators have studied the differential effects of n-3 PUFA intake on plasma lipids and plasma coagulation parameters, particularly platelet and vessel wall composition and function. These studies are carried out, both in experimental animals and in humans, using marine fish and concentrated fish oils.

ANIMAL STUDIES. In rats, when n-3 PUFA or fish oils containing adequate amounts of this PUFA were given as part of diet, significant increases in EPA and DHA levels in platelet lipids were observed. In addition, decreased linoleic acid and AA contents were often reported [11, 12]. The results concerning the effects of n-3 PUFA on platelet aggregation are difficult to explain. In fact, depending on the aggregating agent used, no changes [13, 14] or reductions [15] have been reported in experimental animals. The administration of MaxEPA to rats reduced platelet thromboxane forma-tion and PGI_2 synthesis by vascular tissue [16].

HUMAN STUDIES. Several studies were carried out to evaluate in humans the in vitro and in vivo effects of n-3 PUFA on plasma and cellular lipids. In vitro incorporation of EPA and DHA in washed human platelets results in an inhibition of platelet aggrega-tion induced by several aggregating agents [17]. In the in vivo studies the quantity of n-3 PUFAs ingested daily ranged from 8 to 30 g either with oils isolated mainly from salmon or with MaxEPA, a commercial preparation containing 18% purified EPA and 12% DHA.

In man, the administration of EPA results in the incorporation of this fatty acid in lipids of various cells and tissues, in particular in platelet phospholipids. In fact, an increase of EPA and DHA contents was observed, with a concomitant reduction of AA content [18], leading to a significant increase of the EPA:AA ratio. These modifications of the fatty acid composition of platelet phospholipids are accompanied by a reduction of TXA_2 formation by platelets [19, 20]. Knapp et al. have demon-strated that urinary TXB_2 excretion is greatly reduced in human volunteers following a dietary supplementation with MaxEPA (10 g/day MaxEPA) for 1 month, whereas PGI_2 synthesis was not modified. In the same subjects the urinary excretion of PGI_3 and TXB_3 metabolites was also significantly increased [21].

Regarding platelet aggregation, studies of dietary supplementation with fish oil in normal volunteers have generally reported little or no effect on platelet aggregation induced by several aggregating agents [11, 20, 22]. In particular, the effects of n-3 PUFA appear to be dependent on the amounts of n-3 PUFA in the diet and/or on the stimulus employed to induce platelet aggregation [18, 23].

Effects of Fish Oils on Leukotriene Formation

The metabolism of AA via the lipoxygenase pathway leads in platelets to the formation of 12-hydroxyeicosatetraenoic acid (HETE), a compound which is chemotactic for polymorphonuclear leukocytes and is able to induce smooth-muscle cell proliferation [24, 25]. In leukocytes, AA is metabolized via the 5-lipoxygenase pathway to 5-HETE and leukotriene B_4 (LTB_4), with chemotactic activity, and LTC_4, with vasoconstrictive effects [26, 27].

EPA is a quite good substrate for lipoxygenases and is converted to LTB_5, which is far less active than LTB_4 in affecting neutrophil functions, i.e. aggregation, degranulation and chemokinesis [28].

Dietary supplemention with MaxEPA for 6 weeks to healthy volunteers leads to incorporation of EPA into the membrane lipids of polymorphonuclear leukocytes and monocytes. As a consequence, LTB_4 formation by both cells after calcium ionophore stimulation is decreased. In addition, the LTB_4-mediated chemotaxis and endothelial-cell adherence of neutrophils is significantly reduced [29].

The findings that EPA inhibits LTB_4 production while increasing the formation of LTB_5, which is at least 20-fold less potent in stimulating polymorphonuclear leukocytes than LTB_4, leads to the hypothesis that a diet enriched in EPA may exert anti-inflammatory effects. This hypothesis is also supported by studies which show that changes in fatty acid composition of the diet, and in particular supplementation of EPA, may result in beneficial effects in patients with rheumatoid arthritis [30].

Conclusions

The data reported here on the effects of dietary supplementation with n-3 PUFA indicate that these fatty acids may exert beneficial effects on biochemical and functional parameters of platelets, vessel wall and leukocytes. Thus, a fish oil diet can be useful not only in the treatment of thrombosis and atherosclerosis but also that of inflammation.

More clinical data are still necessary to clarify the effects of fish oil diets. In addition, the potential toxicity of n-3 PUFA should be carefully monitored.

References

1. Hamberg M, Swensson J, Samuelsson B (1975) Thromboxanes: a new group of biologically active compounds derived from prostaglandin endoperoxides. Proc Natl Acad Sci USA 72: 2994–2998

2. Moncada S, Vane JR (1978) Pharmacology and endogenous roles of prostaglandin endoperoxide, thromboxane A_2 and prostaglandin. Pharmacol Rev 30: 293–331
3. Needleman P, Raz A, Minkes MS, Ferrendelli JA, Sprecher H (1979) Triene prostaglandins: prostacyclin and thromboxane biosynthesis and unique biological properties. Proc Natl Acad Sci USA 76: 944–948
4. Fischer S, Weber PC (1983) Thromboxane A_3 (TXA_3) is formed in human platelets after dietary eicosapentaenoic acid (20:5 omega 3). Biochem Biophys Res Comm 16: 1091–1099
5. Spector AA, Kaduce TL, Figard TH et al. (1983) Eicosapentaenoic acid and prostacyclin production by cultured human endothelial cells. J Lip Res 24: 1595–1604
6. Bang HO, Dyerberg J (1980) Lipid metabolism and ischemic heart disease in Greenland Eskimos. In: Draper HH (ed) Advanced nutrition research, vol 3. Plenum, New York, pp 1–22
7. Dyerberg J, Bang HO (1979) Haemostatic function and platelet polyunsaturated fatty acid in Eskimos. Lancet ii: 433–435
8. Kromann N, Green A (1980) Epidemiological studies in the Upernavik district, Greenland. Acta Med Scand 208: 401–406
9. Dyerberg J, Bang HO, Hjorne N (1975) Fatty acid composition of the plasma lipids in Greenland Eskimos. Am J Clin Nutr 28: 958–966
10. Bang HO, Dyerberg J (1980) The bleeding tendency in Greenland Eskimos. Dan Med Bull 27: 202–205
11. Culp BR, Lands WEM, Luchesi BR, Pitt B, Romson J (1980) The effect of dietary supplementation of fish oil on experimental infarction. Prostaglandins 20: 1021–1031
12. Socini A, Galli C, Colombo C, Tremoli E (1983) Fish oil administration as a supplement to a corn oil containing diet affects arterial prostacyclin more than thromboxane formation in the rat. Prostaglandins 25: 693–710
13. Morita I, Saito Y, Chang WC, Murota S (1983) Effects of purified eicosapentaenoic acid or arachidonic acid metabolism in cultured murine aortic smooth muscle cells, vessel walls and platelets. Lipids 1842–1849
14. Bruckner GG, Lokesh B, German B, Kinsella JE (1984) Biosynthesis of prostanoids, tissue fatty acid composition and thrombotic parameters in rats fed diets enriched with docosahexaenoic or eicosapentaenoic acid. Thromb Res 34: 479–497
15. Morisaki N, Shiriomiya M, Matsuoka N et al. (1983) In vivo effects of cis-5,8,11,14,17–20:5 (n-3) and cis-4,7,10,13,16,19–22:6 (n-3) on serum lipoproteins, platelet aggregation and lipid metabolism in the aorta of rats. Tohoku J Exp Med 141: 397–405
16. Hornstra G, Chris-Hazelhof E, Hadderman E et al. (1981) Fish oil feeding lowers thromboxane and prostacyclin production by rat platelet and aorta and does not result in the formation of prostaglandin I_3. Prostaglandins 21: 727–738
17. Croset M, Lagarde M (1986) In vitro incorporation and metabolism of eicosapentaenoic and docosahexaenoic acids in human platelets. Effect on aggregation. Thromb Haemost 56: 57–62
18. Siess W, Scherer B, Bohling B, Roth P, Kurzmann I, Weber PC (1980) Platelet-membrane fatty acids, platelet aggregation, and thromboxane formation during a mackerel diet. Lancet I: 441–444
19. Goodnight SH, Harris WS, Connor WE (1981) The effects of dietary ω-3 fatty acids on platelet composition and function in man: a prospective study. Blood 58: 880–885
20. Von Schacky C, Fisher S, Weber PC (1985) Long-term effects of dietary marine ω-3 fatty acids upon plasma and cellular lipids, platelet function and eicosanoids formation in humans. J Clin Invest 76: 1626–1631
21. Knapp HR, Reilly IAG, Alessandrini P, Fitzgerald GA (1986) In vivo indexes of platelet and vascular function during fish-oil administration in patients with atherosclerosis. N Engl J Med 314: 937–942
22. Terano T, Hirai A, Hamazaki T et al. (1983) Effect of oral administration of highly purified eicosapentaenoic acid on platelet function, blood viscosity and red cell deformability in healthy human subjects. Atherosclerosis 46: 321–326
23. Thorngren M, Gustafson A (1981) Effects of 11-week increase in dietary eicosapentaenoic acid on bleeding time, lipids, and platelet aggregation. Lancet ii: 1190–1193
24. Hamberg M, Samuelsson B (1974) Prostaglandin endoperoxides: novel transformations of arachidonic acid in human platelets. Proc Natl Acad Sci USA 71: 3400–3404

25. Hamberg M (1980) On the mechanism of the oxygenation of arachidonic acid by human platelet lipoxygenase. Biochem Biophys Res Commun 95: 1090–1095
26. Borgeat P, Samuelsson B (1979) Arachidonic acid metabolism in polymorphonuclear leukocytes: effects of ionophore A23187. Proc Natl Acad Sci USA 76: 2148–2152
27. Bjork J, Hedqvist P, Arfors KE (1982) Increase in vascular permeability induced by leukotriene B and the role of polymorphonuclear leukocytes. Inflammation 6: 189–200
28. Terano T, Salmon JA, Higgs GA, Moncada S (1986) Eicosapentaenoic acid as a modulator of inflammation. Biochem Pharmacol 35: 779–785
29. Lee TH, Hoover RL, Williams JD et al. (1985) Effect of dietary enrichment with eicosapentaenoic and docosahexaenoic acids on in vitro neutrophil and monocyte leukotriene generation and neutrophil function. N Engl J Med 312: 1217–1224
30. Kremer JM, Michaelek AV, Lininger L et al. (1985) Effects of manipulation of dietary fatty acids on clinical manifestations of rheumatoid arthritis. Lancet i: 184–187

Oxidative Metabolism of Unsaturated Fatty Acids and Free Radical Formation

J. Bremer, S. Bergseth, and Ø. Spydevold

Our interest in the metabolism of C_{22} fatty acids, both mono- and polyunsaturated, started around 1970. In that year Abdellatif and Vles [1] published their study showing that feeding great amounts of rapeseed oil containing the monounsaturated erucic acid ($C_{22}:1$) to rats caused acute lipidosis of the heart. Later a Canadian group showed that hydrogenated fish oil to some degree had the same effect [2]. The fat infiltration proved to be temporary. If the feeding of these fats is continued the fat infiltration disappears again. Evidently, an adaptation to these diets takes place.

Oxidation of C_{22}-Monounsaturated Acids

To study the oxidation of these long-chain fatty acids we prepared their carnitine esters and tested them as substrates for isolated mitochondria from heart and other tissues. These experiments showed that the C_{22} fatty acids, both mono- and polyunsaturated indeed are poorly oxidized by mitochondria compared with ordinary fatty acids. Also, the presence of these very long-chain fatty acids interferes with the oxidation of the shorter-chain acids, e. g., palmitate [3, 4].

We assume, therefore, that basically the reason for the fat accumulation in the heart, when we feed animals with erucic acid, is its slow oxidation in the mitochondria.

However, the mitochondria experiments gave no explanation for the adaptation phenomenon. Isolated mitochondria from rats adapted for several weeks to these fat diets showed no increased ability to oxidize erucoylcarnitine.

In 1976 Lazarow and deDuve [5] showed that peroxisomes contain a second β-oxidation system for fatty acids, and they showed that this system is induced in the liver of rats fed the hypolipemic drug clofibrate. The fatty acid oxidase of the peroxisomes has hydrogen peroxide as reaction product. The observations of Lazarow and deDuve led us to test whether the peroxisomes are active in the oxidation of the very long-chain fatty acids and whether the adaptation to their presence in the diet was caused by changed peroxisomal activity.

Figure 1 shows that erucic acid is poorly metabolized by isolated hepatocytes from normal rats in comparison with palmitate. However, in hepatocytes from rats adapted to clofibrate diets, the oxidation of erucic acid was increased and about as rapid as the oxidation of palmitate. Esterification was also increased.

Figure 1 also shows that increased amounts of erucic acid were recovered in the cell lipids as shortened products, especially in animals fed clofibrate or hydrogenated fish oil.

H. U. Klör (Ed.)
Lipoprotein Subfractions
Omega-3 Fatty Acids
© Springer-Verlag Berlin Heidelberg 1989

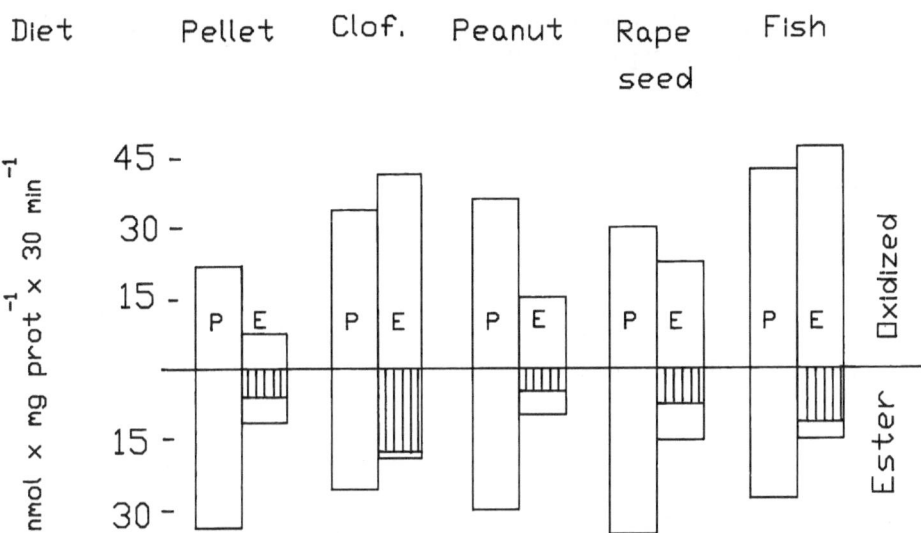

Fig. 1. Comparison of palmitate (P) and erucate (E) metabolism in isolated hepatocytes from rats fed different diets: Low fat pellets (*pellet*), low fat pellets + 0.3% clofibrate (*clof.*), and high fat diets (30% of the calories) with peanut oil (*peanut*) rapeseed oil (*rapeseed*), and partially hydrogenated fish oil (*fish*). The rapeseed oil and the fish oil contained 11.5% C_{22} monounsaturated fatty acids. The isolated cells were incubated with 0.5 mM (16–^{14}C)-palmitate or (14–^{14}C)-erucate for 30 min. The *vertical hatching* indicates erucic acid recovered in the cell lipids as shortened fatty acids

To get further support for the idea that the peroxisomes are involved in the metabolism of these fatty acids we tested the effect of *D*-decanoylcarnitine. This is the unphysiological isomer of the carnitine ester which inhibits the carnitine-dependent mitochondrial fatty acid oxidation, while it has no effect on the carnitine-independent fatty acid oxidation in the peroxisomes.

Addition of *D*-decanoylcarnitine inhibited the oxidation both of palmitate and erucate. However, *D*-decanoylcarnitine gave increased recovery of shortened fatty acids (oleate) from erucate in the cells [6].

Direct measurement of peroxisomal fatty acid oxidation has shown that particularly hydrogenated fish oil and hydrogenated rapeseed oil increased the activity of the peroxisomal β-oxidation enzyme system [7].

These results show that erucate and other C_{22} fatty acids to a great extent depend on the peroxisomes for their normal metabolism. The acids are shortened by one or two β-oxidation cycles in the peroxisomes and then transferred to the mitochondria for complete oxidation. The adaptation to the presence of these fatty acids in the diet is the result mainly of an increased peroxisomal β-oxidation capacity which means an increased shortening capacity. This adaptation also means an increased rate of hydrogen peroxide formation in the tissues. In accordance with these results Foerster et al. [8] have shown in perfused livers that erucic acid increases the formation of hydrogen peroxide. Palmitate had no effect indicating that this acid normally is oxidized almost exclusively in the mitochondria. The role of peroxisomes in the oxidation of the very-long fatty acids (C_{22}–C_{24}) was also confirmed by the detection of accumulated C_{24} fatty acids in the tissues of patients with Zellweger's syndrome. These patients have no peroxisomes in their tissues.

Oxidation of Polyunsaturated Acids

We have investigated whether clofibrate and our high fat diets influence the capacity of the liver to oxidize polyunsaturated fatty acids with up to six double bonds [9]. Figure 2 shows that hepatocytes from rats adapted to clofibrate in the diet have an increased capacity to form ketone bodies, particularly from the polyunsaturated fatty acids. In normal cells ketogenesis from dodecanehexaenoic acid was less than half of that from palmitate, while in hepatocytes from rats fed clofibrate ketogenesis was nearly equal from all the fatty acids tried, including dodecanehexaenoic acid. Ketogenesis from this acid was nearly threefold increased by feeding clofibrate. The same high ketogenesis from long-chain polyunsaturated fatty acids was found in hepatocytes from rats fed hydrogenated fish oil. Hagve and Christophersen [10] tested the importance of peroxisomes in the metabolism of different [1–^{14}C]-labelled unsaturated fatty acids in hepatocytes by measuring the effect of D-decanoylcarnitine. Their results suggest that the role of the peroxisomes varies extensively for the different acids. Thus, the oxidation of oleate and arachidonate (C_{20}:4) were strongly

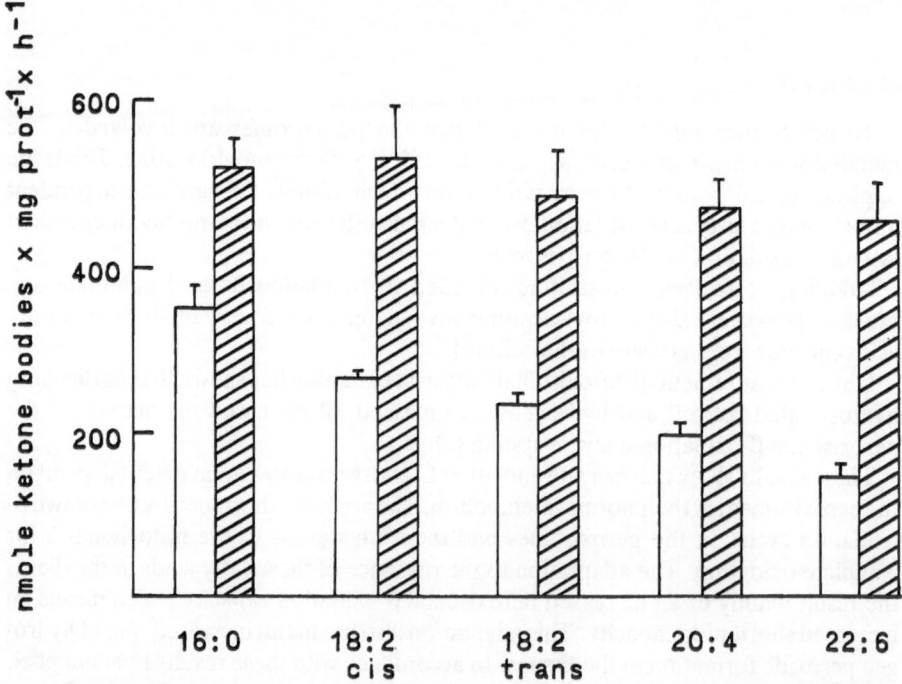

Fig. 2. Ketogenesis from palmitate (16:0) and different unsaturated fatty acids in isolated hepatocytes from rats fed low fat pellets (*open columns*) and low fat pellets + 0.3% clofibrate (*hatched columns*). The cells were incubated with the different fatty acids in a concentration of 2 mM

inhibited by D-decanoylcarnitine, while the oxidation of eicosapetenoate was less inhibited and the oxidation of adrenic acid (C_{22}:4) was nearly unaffected [10]. These results show that peroxisomal oxidation is important in the metabolism of some polyunsaturated fatty acids, e.g., adrenic acid. High levels in the diet induce peroxisomal β-oxidation activity, and they are peroxisomal substrates which thus will increase the production of hydrogen peroxide in the tissues.

Dealing with the Double Bonds

In experiments with different inhibitors of mitochondrial fatty acid oxidation we were intrigued by finding that 4-pentenoate had lost completely its inhibitory effect on fatty acid oxidation in hepatocytes from clofibrate-fed rats [11]. The β-oxidation of 4-pentenoate will give pent-2,4-dienoyl-CoA. This reminded us of the work by Kunau and Dommes [12] who detected the enzyme 2,4-dienoyl-CoA reductase. The 2,4-dienoyl-CoA esters with their conjugated double bonds are poorly hydrated by crotonase in the β-oxidation reaction sequence, and Kunau and Dommes suggested that their enzyme, converting the 2,4-dienoyl-CoA ester to a 3-enoyl-CoA by reduction with NADPH, take part in the oxidation of unsaturated fatty acids with double bonds at equal-numbered positions. Thus, the oxidation of these fatty acids should paradoxically depend on a reduction step.

Because of the insensitivity of hepatocytes from clofibrate-fed rats to pentenoate, we measured the activity of the 2,4-dienoyl-CoA reductase in these hepatocytes and found a five fold increase [11]. The increase of this enzyme prevents the accumulation of the toxic 2,4-pentdienoyl-CoA in the mitochondria because it is rapidly converted to the easily metabolizable 3-pentenoyl-CoA. Later we found that diets high in fish oil or in some hydrogenated fats also increased the activity of this enzyme (Fig. 3) [10]. The 2,4-dienoyl-CoA reductase is present both in the mitochondria and in the peroxisomes [12]. Oxidation of fatty acids with equal-numbered double bonds therefore requires NADPH also in the peroxisomes. It is paradoxical that hydrogenated fats where most of the double bonds have been removed are as strong inducers of the 2,4-dienoyl-CoA reductase as are the unhydrogenated fats. The hydrogenated fats were also more efficient in the induction of the peroxisomal β-oxidation enzymes. Apparently the chain length of the fatty acids is more important than the presence of double bonds in the induction of all these enzymes in vivo.

We have also tested the inducing effect of fatty acids on peroxisomal activity in a hepatoma cell culture (Fig. 4). In such experiments the specificity of the fatty acids as inducers proved to be different. The optimal chain length of saturated fatty acids was C_{14} (myristic acid). Longer-chain fatty acids were less efficient. Introduction of double bonds increased the inducing effect. The effects of stearate, linolate, and linolenate increased in that order (Fig. 4).

Significance of Increased Hydrogen Peroxide Formation

In prolonged feeding of rapeseed oil with a high content of erucic acid, the lipidosis of the heart disappears after a couple of weeks. However, such feeding may lead to focal

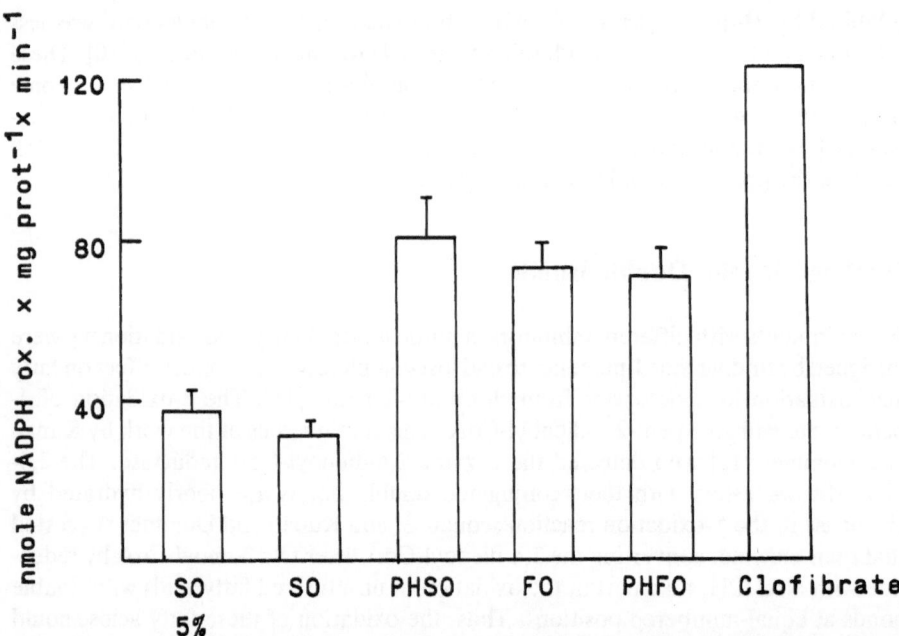

Fig. 3. The activity of 2,4-dienoyl-CoA reductase in the liver of rats fed different fat diets: 5% soybean oil (*SO*), 25% soybean oil (*SO*), 25% partially hydrogenated soybean oil (*PHSO*) 25% fish oil (*FO*), 25% partially hydrogenated fish oil (*PHFO*), or low fat pellets + 0.3% clofibrate

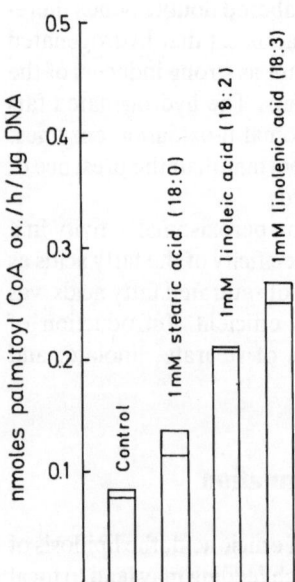

Fig. 4. Induction of peroxisomal fatty acid oxidation by fatty acids in hepatoma cells in vitro. Morris hepatoma cells 7800 C_1 [19] were grown in Ham's F 10 medium with 10% horse serum and 3% calf serum in the absence or presence of 1 m*M* fatty acid for 3 days (two parallels)

necrosis and fibrosis in the heart [14]. Induction of peroxisomes in the heart by hydrogenated fish oil has been demonstrated [15] but it is not known whether the increased hydrogen peroxide load contributes to the observed tissue damage.

It has repeatedly been shown that high fat diets can promote cancer development and different mechanisms have been suggested. So-called prooxidant states, involving active oxygen radicals seem to promote tumor development [16], and Reddy and coworkers [17] have suggested that increased hydrogen peroxide formation due to peroxisome proliferation may explain the cancer-promotion effects of some hypolipemic, peroxisome-proliferating drugs, like clofibrate. Lillehaug et al. [18] have shown that some peroxisome-proliferating drugs show such promotor effects in mouse embryo fibroblasts in tissue culture, but it is still unknown whether peroxisome-inducing fatty acids have such effects. Peroxidation of unsaturated fatty acids is assumed to contribute to pro-oxidant states in tissues. Peroxisome proliferation and peroxisomal β-oxidation is an additional mechanism by which certain high-fat diets can increase peroxide formation in the tissues.

References

1. Abdellatif AMM, Vles RO (1970) Pathological effects of dietary rapeseed oil in rats. Nutr. Metab 12: 285–295
2. Beare-Rogers JL, Nera EA, Craig BM (1972) Accumulation of cardiac fatty acids in rats fed synthesized oils containing C-22 fatty acids. Lipids 7: 46–50
3. Christophersen BO, Bremer J (1972) Carnitine esters of unsaturated fatty acids. Preparation and some aspects of their metabolism. Biochim Biophys Acta 260: 515–526
4. Christophersen BO, Bremer J (1972) Erucic acid. Inhibitor of fatty acid oxidation in heart. Biochim Biophys Acta 280: 506–514
5. Lazarow PB, de Duve C (1976) Fatty acyl-CoA oxidizing system in rat liver peroxisomes. Enhancement by clofibrate, a hypolipidemic drug. Proc Natl Acad Sci 73: 2043–2046
6. Christiansen RZ, Christiansen EN, Bremer J (1979) Stimulation of erucate metabolism in isolated rat hepatocytes by rapeseed oil and hydrogenated marine oil containing diets. Biochim Biophys Acta 573: 417–429
7. Neat CE, Thomassen MS, Osmundsen H (1980) Induction of peroxisomal β-oxidation in rat liver by high fat diets. Biochem J 186: 369–371
8. Foerster EC, Fährenkemper T, Rabe U, Graf P, Sies H (1981) Peroxisomal fatty acid oxidation as detected by H_2O_2 in intact perfused rat liver. Biochem J 196: 705–712
9. Bergseth S, Christiansen EN, Bremer J (1986) The Effect of Feeding Fish Oils and Clofibrate on the Ketogenesis from Long Chain Fatty Acids in Hepatocytes. Lipids 21: 508–514
10. Hagve TA, Christophersen BO (1986) Evidence for retroconversion of adrenic acid (22:4(n-6)) and docosahexaenoic acid (22:6(n-3)) in isolated liver cells. Biochim Biophys Acta 875: 165–173
11. Borrebæk B, Osmundsen H, Bremer J (1980) In vivo induction of 4-enoyl-CoA reductase by clofibrate in liver mitochondria and its effect on Pent-4-enoate metabolism. Biochem. Biophys Res Commun 93: 1173–1180
12. Kunau WH, Dommes P (1981) Degradation of unsaturated fatty acids. Identification of intermediates in degradation of Cis-4-d-ecenoyl-CoA by extracts of beef liver mitochondria. Eur J Biochem 91: 533–544
13. Dommes V, Baumgart C, Kunau WH (1981) Degradation of unsaturated fatty acids in peroxisomes. Existence of a 2,4-dienoyl-CoA reductase pathway. J Biol Chem 256: 8259–8262
14. Roine P, Uksila E, Teir H, Rapola J (1960) Histopathological changes in rats and pigs fed rapeseed oil. Z Ernährungswiss 1: 118–124
15. Norseth J, Thomassen MS (1983) Stimulation of microperoxisomal β-oxidation in rat heart by high fat diets. Biochim Biophys Acta 751: 312–320

106   J. Bremer et al.

16. Cerutti PA (1985) Prooxidant states and tumor promotion. Science 227: 375–381
17. Reddy JK, Warren JR, Reddy MK, Lalwani ND (1982) Hepatic and Renal Effects of Peroxisome Proliferators: Biological Implications. Ann NY Academy of Sciences 386: 81–110
18. Lillehaug JR, Aarsæther N, Berge RK, Male R (1986) Peroxisome proliferators show tumor promoting but no direct transforming activity in vitro. Int J Cancer 37: 97–100
19. Richardson UI, Snodgrass PJ, Nuzum CT, Tashjian AH (1973) Establishment of a clonal strain of hepatoma cells which maintain in culture 5 enzymes of urea cycle. J Cell Physiol 83: 141–150

Omega-3 Fatty Acids and Hemostasis

M. Lagarde, M. Croset, and E. Véricel

Interactions between platelets and vascular endothelial cells play a key role in hemostasis and particularly primary hemostasis. In this context, the metabolism of arachidonic acid is believed to be an important point. When platelets are triggered with aggregating agents like collagen or thrombin, arachidonic acid is liberated from membrane phospholipids and then subsequently oxygenated by two pathways. One of these pathways is the cyclooxygenase which leads to PGH_2, readily converted into TXA_2. Both compounds are pro-aggregatory molecules and have also a vasocontracting activity. TXA_2 is quite labile and it is degraded into TXB_2 which is not active. PGH_2 is also transformed into small amounts of primary prostaglandins PGE_2, F2α, and D2. The second pathway is the lipoxygenase one, which catalyzes specifically the oxygenation of carbon 12, leading to 12-hydroperoxy-eicosatetraenoic acid (12-HPETE) or 12-hydroperoxy-arachidonic acid, which is further reduced into its 12 hydroxy products, 12-HETE, by a glutathione-dependent peroxydase. PGH_2 of platelet origin may also be transformed into prostacyclin (PGI_2), a very potent anti-aggregating and vasodilating agent produced by vascular endothelium. PGI_2 may also be formed from endogenous arachidonic acid when liberated from endothelial phospholipids by specific agonists like bradykinin or thrombin.

Various polyunsaturated fatty acids of nutritional interest may alter this metabolism in different ways. One way is to affect the oxygenation of arachidonic acid, a second way is to affect cell functions through their own metabolites. Among these, two fatty acids found in substantial amounts in fish fat are of particular interest. They are eicosapentaenoic acid (EPA) or 20:5 ω3 and docosahexaenoic acid (DHA) or 22:6 ω3. EPA is closely related to arachidonic acid, with an additional double bound between carbon 17 and 18. In contrast, DHA is quite different; it has two additional carbons and six double bounds at different positions [4, 7, 10, 13, 16, 19]. This difference will not allow it to compete with arachidonic acid oxygenation as EPA does.

Concerning the dietary approach, numerous studies have shown that fish fat consumption reduces platelet aggregability and thromboxane formation, presumably due to EPA. However, since fish fat contains large amounts of DHA, this acid can account for the inhibition observed. Most studies relate to the intake of 2–10 g/day of EPA, which results in replacing part of cell arachidonic acid by EPA. These high doses may induce some side effects. In addition, most of the studies concern intake of crude fish oil, which includes a rather high amount of saturated fat. EPA is poorly oxygenated into thromboxane A_3, which is a weak aggregating agent. It inhibits competitively 20:4 ω6 oxygenation in platelets and decreases 20:4 ω6 lipid contents, then reducing TXA_2 formation. It also generates PGD_3, which shares the anti-

H. U. Klör (Ed.)
Lipoprotein Subfractions
Omega-3 Fatty Acids
© Springer-Verlag Berlin Heidelberg 1989

aggregating activity of PGD_2, and could be involved in the anti-aggregating effect of EPA. Finally, its lipoxygenase product (12-OH-20:5) antagonizes PGH_2/TXA_2-induced aggregation, even more potently than 12-HETE, the lipoxygenase product of arachidonic acid. In endothelial cells, EPA is converted into PGI_3, which is a prostacyclin-lik molecule, and induces only a moderate decrease of prostacyclin formation.

As far as the inflammation processes are concerned, EPA is converted into peptidoleukotrienes (LTC_5 and D_5), but until now, we do not know anything about the biological activity of such compounds. It decreases LTB_4 formation, and it is also converted into LTB_5, which is at least five times less chemotactic than LTB_4.

Finally, it reduces platelet activating factor generation in polymorphonuclear neutrophiles.

Much less is known concerning DHA, although it is assumed to be associated with EPA in fish oil-induced platelet inhibition. It is not converted into prostanoids, and it is a poor substrate of animal lipoxygenases.

Our own experience, relating to fatty acids from fish oil, concerns the intake of small amounts of pure EPA. First we used an arginin salt of EPA. For 2 months 50 mg/day of EPA were given to insulin-dependent diabetics or 150 mg/day for 1 month to elderly people, both populations being known to have hyperactive platelets. In both cases, platelet aggregability was decreased without any alteration of plasma and platelet fatty acid profiles [1, 2]. The inhibition of aggregation could be observed when collagen, thrombin, or adrenaline, but not exogenous 20:4 ω6, was used as the aggregating agent. This suggests that EPA intake was able to inhibit platelet aggregation when induced by an agent requiring the liberation of endogenous arachidonic acid. Therefore, we undertook a new experiment with elderly people with a more physiological form of EPA. Eight elderly people received 100 mg/day of EPA in a triglyceride form, (1,3-dioctanoyl, 2-eicosapentaenoyl-glycerol) for 2 months. Another eight elderly people received a placebo in a double-blind, randomized study. A number of tests were used, including platelet aggregability, the oxygenation of endogenous arachidonic acid, and the fatty acid profiles of plasma and platelet lipid stores. We also measured plasma and platelet tocopherols. Among these various tests, only two gave different results after EPA intake. They were platelet aggregability, which was significantly decreased as in our previous studies, and platelet tocopherols (α and γ), which were significantly increased. After EPA, platelet tocopherols were increased to values very close to those of platelets from young adults.

We conclude that low intake of EPA decreases platelet aggregation in a prethrombotic state like aging, without affecting the stimulated metabolism of arachidonic acid, nor the plasma and the platelet fatty acid compositions. Platelet vitamin E, which is significantly reduced in elderly people compared with young adults, was significantly increased to normal levels. We may then suggest that hyperaggregability of platelets from elderly people might be decreased in reducing their peroxide tone.

We have also performed some in vitro experiments with DHA. It was preincorporated into platelets after being precoated onto free fatty acid albumin. Under these conditions, most of the fatty acid was incorporated into phospholipids. Then platelets were rewashed and used for further experiments. The aggregability of DHA-rich platelets was compared with that of control platelets as well as platelets preenriched with EPA in a similar way. The aggregation was induced by thrombin, collagen, or the stable analogue of TXA_2, U-46619. There was a significant decrease of the aggregability of EPA- or DHA-rich platelets, whatever the aggregating agent used. Interestingly, DHA was even more potent than EPA for inhibiting the aggregation. In using radio-labeled fatty acids instead of unlabeled ones, we were able to measure the platelet metabolism of preenriched fatty acid. When platelets were stimulated by thrombin or the calcium ionophore A 23187, there was a significant decrease of arachidonic acid in phospholipids, and a significant formation of its lipoxygenase product and TXB_2. The metabolic pattern of preincorporated EPA was quite similar, with a significant decrease of EPA in total phospholipids and a substantial formation of its lipoxygenese product (even higher than from arachidonic acid), and a small formation of TXB_3. The situation was entirely different with DHA. When DHA was preincorporated into platelets, their stimulation by phospholipase inducers did not induce any decrease of liberation of this acid from phospholipids.

The detailed metabolism of each fatty acid in phospholipid subclasses under thrombin or ionophore stimulation was also different as far as DHA is concerned. The pattern of EPA appeared quite superimposable on that of arachidonic acid, the main features being a decrease in both phosphatidylinositol and phosphatidylcholine and a weak reacylation into phosphatidyl-ethanolamine, at least for arachidonic acid. In contrast and unexpected from the results obtained with total phospholipids, one-fourth of DHA incorporated into phosphatidylcholine was liberated and reacylated into phosphatidylethanolamine in a reciprocal way.

We conclude that DHA preincorported into platelet lipid stores is even more potent than EPA for inhibiting platelet aggregation. Whereas EPA is liberated from phospholipids and efficiently oxygenated by platelet cyclooxygenase and lipoxygenase, DHA is not freed. However, it is substantially transfered from phosphatidylcholine to phosphatidylethanolamine.

In summary, we can say that the inhibition of platelet aggregation by EPA does not necessarily require the replacement of endogenous arachidonic acid and the inhibition of arachidonic acid oxygenation. Small amounts of EPA might act in modulating the peroxide tone of the cell. On the other hand, DHA is even more potent than EPA for inhibiting platelet aggregation but the respective mechanisms for such inhibitions appear entirely different.

References

1. Velardo B, Lagarde M, Guichardant M, Dechavanne M, Beylot M, Sautot G, Berthezene F (1982) Decrease of platelet activity after intake of small amounts of eicosapentaenoic acid in diabetics. Thrombos Haemostas 38: 344
2. Driss F, Véricel E, Lagarde M, Dechavanne M, Darcet P (1984) Inhibition of platelet aggregation and thromboxane synthesis after intake of small amount of eicosapentaenoic acid in the elderly. Thrombos Res 36: 389–396

The Effects of Omega-3 Fatty Acids in Multiple Sclerosis: 2-Year-Results

J. M. French, D. Bates, S. A. Hawkins, A. D. Smith,
and R. H. S. Thompson

Introduction

It has been noted that Multiple Sclerosis was more prevalent in more northern and colder climates than in the more southern and warmer countries. In 1950 Swank [1] first proposed an association between dietary intake and the incidence of Multiple sclerosis, – countries such as Canada, the United Kingdom and other countries in Europe recording dietary fat intake two to three times that in Cuba, Turkey and Italy. The former group of countries had a high incidence of Multiple Sclerosis, the latter a low incidence. This association was reinforced when the fluctuations in fat intake before, during and after World War II mirrored changes in the incidence of Multiple Sclerosis throughout Europe. Sinclair [2] later suggested that the link might rather be a deficient intake of polyunsaturated fatty acids (PUFA), and this theory was borne out by Thompson and coworkers [3, 4, 5] who found reduced levels of linoleate in the serum, erythrocytes and lymphocytes of patients with Multiple Sclerosis. It was known that the addition of linoleate [6] to the diet of healthy people rapidly increases their serum levels, and in 1973 Millar et al. [7] reported the results of a double-blind trial using sunflower seed oil as the supplement in a treated group and oleic acid in a control group. They found that relapses were less severe and of shorter duration in the treated group. This finding was confirmed by Bates et al. [8] in Newcastle, but not by a subsequent report from Canada by Paty et al. [9].

The exact role of polyunsaturated fats in Multiple Sclerosis is unknown. Their transformation into prostaglandins and an effect on the immune system may be one mode of action; Fig. 1 illustrates the formation of the different series of prostaglandins derived from the fats of the omega-3 and the omega-6 classes. Eicosapentaenoic acid is plentiful in fish body oil, and it was decided to undertake a dietary trial using this acid as the supplement.

The Trial

The trial was double-blind. One group received capsules containing 0.5 g MaxEPA oil, the total daily dose providing approximately 3 g oil of the omega-3 series, the other group identical capsules containing 72% oleic acid. Both groups were given identical dietary advice to increase their intake of omega-6 polyunsaturated fats and

H. U. Klör (Ed.)
Lipoprotein Subfractions
Omega-3 Fatty Acids
© Springer-Verlag Berlin Heidelberg 1989

PUFA metabolism (n-6 : n-3)

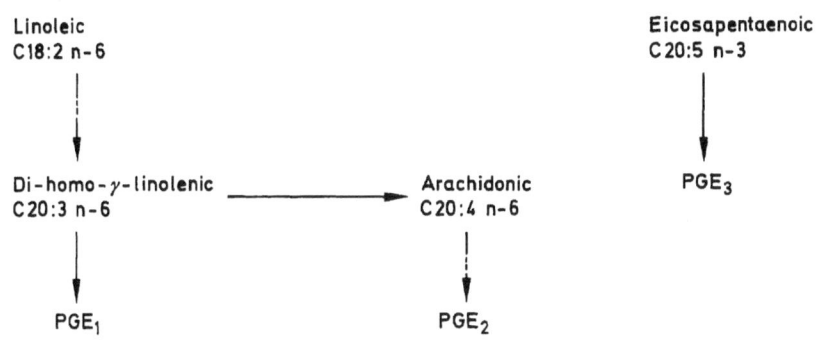

Fig. 1. Prostaglandin production – PGE$_1$, PGE$_2$ and PGE$_3$

reduce their intake of animal fat. It was necessary to take 20 capsules daily to attain the required level.

Patients aged 16–45 years were recruited from three centres: Belfast, London and Newcastle upon Tyne. All patients had clinically definite Multiple Sclerosis by the criteria of MacDonald and Halliday [7], and all had the acute relapsing form of the disease. Only patients with a Kurtzke disability score less than or equal to 6 were admitted, and all patients had suffered at least one relapse in the previous 24 months. On entry to the trial the patients were stratified by age and sex and randomised to the treatment or the control group. A total of 312 patients were entered: 74 in Belfast, 43 in London and 195 in Newcastle. Of these, 101 were male and 211 female – reflecting the greater prevalence of the disease in females. Table 1 shows that no significant differences existed between the two groups with respect to sex distribution, age, duration of disease, severity of disease or HLA status. It is, however, of interest to note, that the level of DR2 in the normal population is in the region of 25%–30%.

Patients were seen at entry and at 3-month intervals, when their Kurtzke disability status was evaluated and a history of relapses noted. Also, at admission and at 6-month intervals fasting blood was collected and fatty acids in the serum subsequently

Table 1. Patient's characteristics at entry to the trial

	Treatment	Control
Number	155	157
Male	53	48
Female	102	109
Age (years) (mean ± SD)	34.0 ± 6.6	33.7 ± 6.3
Duration (years) (mean ± SD)	6.5 ± 4.4	6.6 ± 4.6
K (mean ± SD)	2.6 ± 1.6	2.5 ± 1.6
HLA status		
A3	38.0%	35.8%
B7	45.8%	40.5%
DR2	51.8%	51.0%

Table 2. Serum fatty acid levels

	Linoleic		Arachidonic		Eicosapen taenoic		Docosahexaenoic	
Time	T	C	T	C	T	C	T	C
Entry	34.3	35.3	6.32	6.38	0.87	0.76	2.17	2.16
6 months	35.2	37.6	5.74	6.16	5.18	0.70	4.79	2.03
2 years	35.1	38.2	5.53	6.75	5.89	0.71	4.95	1.96

(T, Treatment (n-3, n-6); C, Control (n-6).
The values represent the amount of each fatty acid as a percentage of the total fatty acid analysed.
Standard errors are in all cases less than 5%

analysed at the Courtauld Institute in London. A cohort of patients from Newcastle and Belfast provided samples of adipose tissue, and these were analysed at the International Institute of Human Nutrition, Oxfordshire. Table 2 illustrates the fatty acid levels in the two groups and the rapid increase of omega-3 fatty acids in the treated group. It should be noted that the level of omega-6 fatty acids in the treated group remained unchanged despite dietary advice, and that the level of arachidonic acid was reduced considerably. Individual patient profiles indicated a very high level of compliance. Results from the, analysis of adipose tissue samples confirmed the increase of omega-3 fatty acids in the treated group but this was not achieved until later in the trial, i.e. after 18–24 months.

Results

Of the 312 patients, 292 completed the 2-year period of the trial. At this stage patients had a detailed neurological examination and the Kurtzke disability score was assessed. There was no difference in outcome between the three centres; Table 3 shows the outcome for the total trial population. One patient died during the 2-year period, and a further 19 were lost to follow-up either due to voluntary withdrawal or because they had moved to another area of the country.

In the treated group 51% of patients remained the same or improved, i.e. their Kurtzke disability score remained unaltered or improved by 1 or more points. In the control group 41.4% improved or remained unchanged. When patients whose Kurtzke disability score was less than or equal to 2 at entry were analysed separately,

Table 3. Outcome at two years

	Treatment (n-3, n-6)		Control (n-6)	
	n	(%)	n	(%)
Same/better	79	(51.0)	65	(41.4)
Worse	66	(42.6)	82	(52.2)
Withdrawn	9	(5.8)	10	(6.4)
Dead	1	(0.6)	0	(0.0)
Total	155	(100.0)	157	(100.0)

the proportion in the treated group who improved or remained the same rose to 58.8%, compared to 45.6% in the control group. None of these values attain statistical significance between the two groups at the 5% level. Duration and severity of relapses also showed a trend in favour of the treated group, but the figures did not reach statistical significance at 5%.

Discussion

Previous trials [7, 8] using PUFA of the omega-6 series as supplement have shown benefit to patients in treated groups with respect to severity and duration of relapses, and where patients with disease of mild disability and short duration were studied, overall outcome was also improved. In the trial described above a statistically significant difference at the 5% level was not achieved; however, in view of the serum fatty acid levels (Table 2) obtained it must be noted that the effect of omega-3 fatty acid supplementation in the treated group negated the effect of the dietary advice of high omega-6 fatty acid intake. In all patients studied, more benefit accrued in the treated patients that in the control patients.

Multiple Sclerosis is a disease known to have periods of long remission with or without therapy. It is unlikely, however, that these spontaneous improvements would occur only in the treated group rather than being equally distributed between the two groups. There is no known cure for Multiple Sclerosis, and in the absence of such it would seem realistic on the evidence, however slim, to recommend to patients that they increase their omega-6 PUFA and increase their omega-3 PUFA either by eating fatty fish such as herring, mackerel or salmon or by taking a daily supplement of fish oil concentrate such as MaxEPA.

Summary

Between 1981 and 1986, 312 ambulant patients from Belfast, London and Newcastle upon Tyne took part in a double-blind controlled trial. The patients were randomly allocated to treatment and control groups, and all were given dietary advice to increase their intake of omega-6 polyunsaturated fatty acid. The treatment group received omega-3 fatty acid supplementation in the form of 20 capsules per day while the control group received 20 identical capsules containing olive oil. Patients were followed for 3–5 years and the results assessed in terms of overall change in Kurtzke disability status scale and number and severity of relapses. Compliance was monitored at regular intervals by estimation of serum fatty acids. The results showed no significant difference in overall outcome at the 5% level though in each category analysed there was less deterioration in patients taking omega-3 oils ($p = 0.07$).

Acknowledgements. The authors would like to thank the Multiple Sclerosis Society of Great Britain and Northern Ireland, who supplied the funding for this research, and also Marfleet Refining Company, who supplied the capsules for both groups.

We would also like to thank the following participants in the trial: N.E.F. Cartlidge, M.J. Jackson, S. Nightingale, D.A. Shaw, S. Smith, E. Woo, J.H.D. Millar*, J. Belin**, D.M. Conroy**, S.K. Gill**, M. Sidey**, M. Gale***, H.M. Sinclair***
  * Department of Neurology, The University of Newcastle upon Tyne,
    Department of Medicine, The Queen's University of Belfast
 ** The National Hospital, Queen Square, London
*** International Institute of Human Nutrition, Sutton Courtenay

References

1. Swank RL (1950) Multiple Sclerosis: a correlation of its incidence with dietary fat. Am J Med Sci 220: 421–430
2. Sinclair HM (1956) Deficiency of essential fatty acids and atherosclerosis. Lancet 381–383
3. Baker RWR, Thompson RHS, Zilkha KJ (1964) Serum fatty acids in Multiple Sclerosis. J Neurol Neurosurg Psychiatry 27: 408–414
4. Baker RWR, Sanders H, Thompson RHS, Zilkha KJ (1965) Serum cholesterol linoleate levels in Multiple Sclerosis. J Neurol Neurosurg Psychiatry 28: 212–217
5. Gul S, Smith AD, Thompson RHS, Payling Wright H, Zilkha KJ (1970) Fatty acid composition of phospholipids from platelets and erythrocytes in Multiple Sclerosis. J Neurol Neurosurg Psychiatry 33: 506–510
6. Belin J, Pettet N, Smith AD, Thompson RHS, Zilkha KJ (1971) Linoleate metabolism in Multiple Sclerosis. J Neurol Neurosurg Psychiatry 34: 25–29
7. Millar JHD, Zilkha KJ, Langman MJS, Payling Wright H, Smith AD, Belin J, Thompson RHS (1973) Double-blind trial of linoleate supplementation of the diet in Multiple Sclerosis. Brit Med J [Clin Res] 1: 765–768
8. Bates D, Fawcett PRW, Shaw DA, Weightman D (1978) Polyunsaturated fatty acids in treatment of acute remitting Multiple Sclerosis. Brit Med J [Clin Res] 2: 1390–1391
9. Paty DW, Cousin HK, Read S, Adlakha K (1978) Linoleic acid in Multiple Sclerosis: failure to show any therapeutic benefit. Acta neurol Scand 58: 53–58

Omega-3 Fatty Acids, Autoimmunity, and Diabetes

Th. Linn

There are essentially three ways autoimmunity may develop. Cytotoxic cells which are functionally deleted by the immune system under normal circumstances are transformed into active cells by an unknown event. Another mechanism is the interaction of cytotoxic cells with cross reactive antigens, e. g. drugs or virus similar to autoantigens. A third pathway to autoimmune mediated destruction is, that cross-reactive antigens are immobilized on target cell membranes.

Autoimmune diseases are basically separated in two different categories, organ-specific diseases and non organ-specific diseases. Juvenile diabetes is an example for an organ-specific autoimmune disease, while rheumatoid arthritis represents a non organ-specific disease. New Zealand Black mice are known to be a model for human lupus erythematosus. In a study undertaken by Prickett et al. [1] these mice were fed fish oil or a beef tallow diet. The fish oil fed group had a longer survival time and decreased extent of renal disease compared with the beef tallow fed group. Moreover, a reduction of the serum titre of DNA antibodies was described. In a placebo-controlled cross-over trial [2] patients with rheumatoid arthritis were treated for a 14-week period either with fish oil or placebo. A number of clinical variables was studied, for instance time to fatigue and tender joints. A significant improvement was found for the fish oil group, maintained for about 4 weeks after stoppage of treatment.

Figure 1 shows inflammation of an islet of Langerhans after chemical induction of immune-mediated diabetic disease by multiple subdiabetogenic doses of streptozocin. Figure 2 demonstrates increased class two antigen expression on vascular endothelium of islets of Langerhans prior to the development of a lymphocytic infiltrate. Class two antigen molecules are genetically determined by the major histocompatibility complex and are located on cell membranes. They are regular structures on immunocompetent cells, such as macrophages and lymphocytes, but they are also present on vascular endothelium, and they are correlated to a state of functional activity in these cells.

There is a 100-fold difference of diabetes incidence between Greenland Eskimos and Western societes. In this connection we have observed that diets greatly enriched with fish oil up to 20% of calorie content result in the incorporation of eicosapentaenoic acid (EPA) into the phospholipid fraction of islets of Langerhans. However, there have been reports that the cells of the immune system behave differently. Some seem to incorporate EPA and some do not. It is not fully understood whether fish oil treatment inhibits the production of arachidonic acid metabolites on the phospholipase level or whether there is some direct effect of omega-3 polyunsaturated fatty acids on the cyclooxygenase system in immunocompetent cells. It is well known that PGE_2 produced by macrophages inhibits the secretion of interleukins. Probably more

H. U. Klör (Ed.)
Lipoprotein Subfractions
Omega-3 Fatty Acids
© Springer-Verlag Berlin Heidelberg 1989

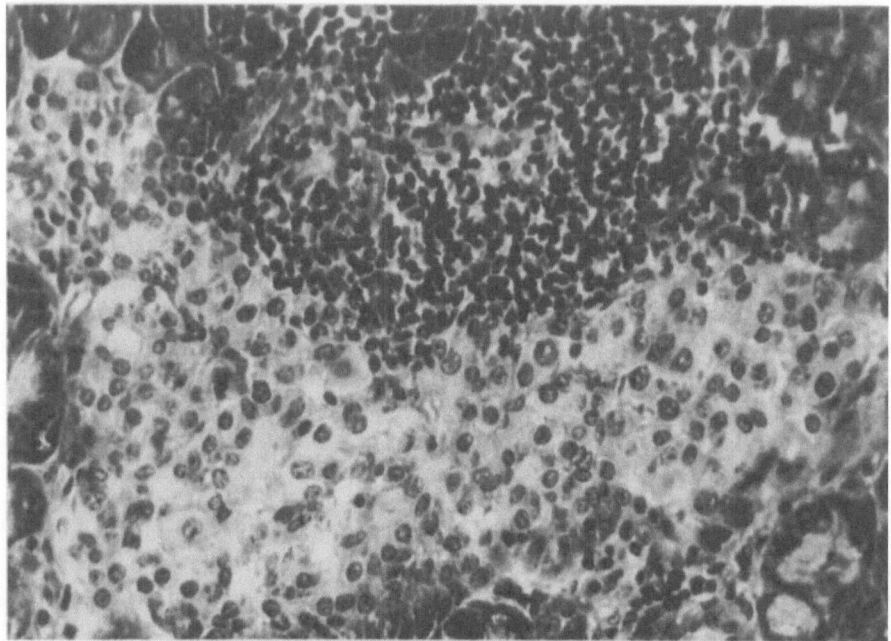

Fig. 1. Lymphocytic infiltration of islet of Langerhans ("insulitis") 2 weeks after diabetes induction with 5 × 40 mg streptozocin per kg and day

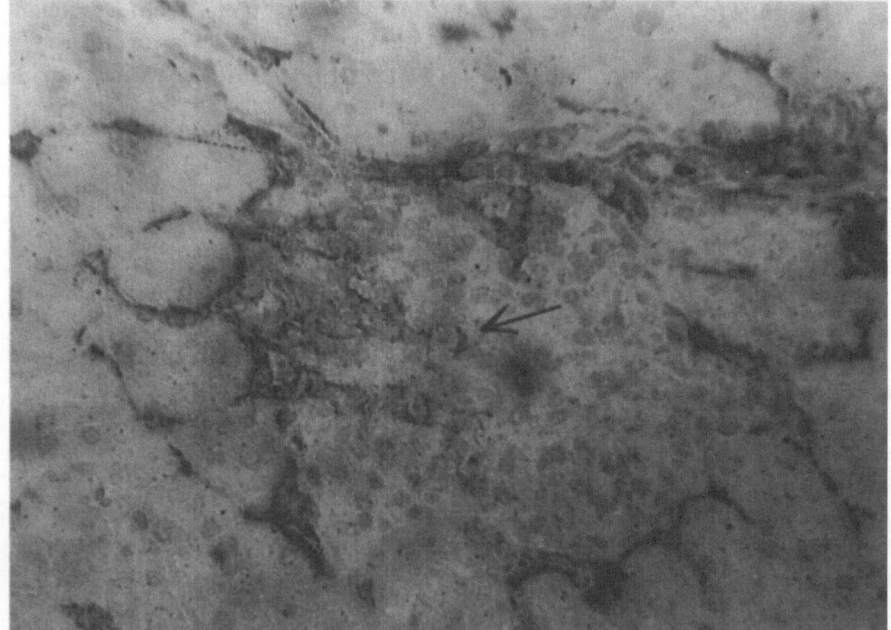

Fig. 2. Increased class two antigen expression on endothelia 3 days after diabetes induction. *Black spots* mark small vessels in the periphery and especially the ductular region of an islet arrow. Staining with monoclonal antibody peroxidase-antiperoxidase; magnification × 450

prostaglandins will be detected that can modulate feedback mechanisms in cell-to-cell interaction. EPA is a better substrate for lipoxygenases than it is for cyclooxygenases. Therefore leukotriene metabolism should be studied. Leukotriene B_4 is the most potent chemotactic agent, whereas the omega-3 derivative leukotriene B_5 is biologically 30 times less potent. Chemotactic responses to a triggering event take place in all cellular immune reactions, including the delayed-type hypersensitivity reaction. Immunocompetent cells with cytotoxic activity directed against antigen carrying cells infiltrate the target tissue via blood vessels destroying their target cells by secretion of cytotoxic lymphokines or by phagocytosis. The morphological correlative of these mechanisms is an inflammatory infiltrate consisting mainly of lymphocytes. During our studies for the past 4 years we have been interested in the lymphocyte infiltrate of islets termed insulitis, which is characteristic for the development of human type I diabetes.

Streptozocin given as a single high dose is cytotoxic to beta cells. When streptozocin is applied in the form of multiple subdiabetogenic doses, blood glucose rises slowly and insulitis is found after 7 to 10 days. This process is sex- and strain-dependent in mice. In C57B16 mice beta cell cytotoxic lymphocytes circulate in the blood as well as islet cell antibodies. These phenomena cannot be found when a single high dose of streptozocin is administered.

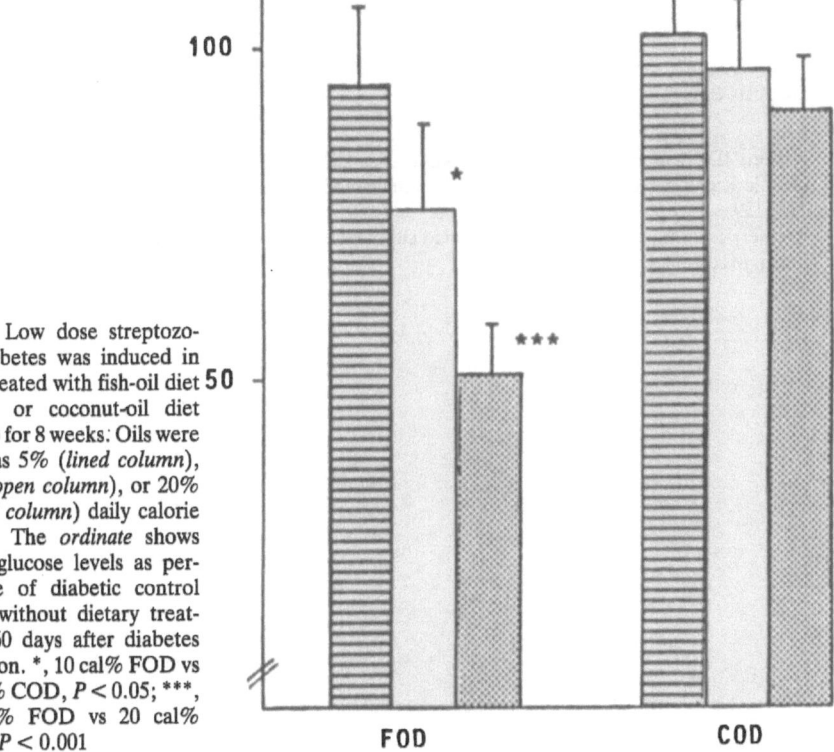

Fig. 3. Low dose streptozocin diabetes was induced in mice treated with fish-oil diet (*FOD*) or coconut-oil diet (*COD*) for 8 weeks. Oils were given as 5% (*lined column*), 10% (*open column*), or 20% (*dotted column*) daily calorie intake. The *ordinate* shows blood glucose levels as percentage of diabetic control group without dietary treatment 60 days after diabetes induction. *, 10 cal% FOD vs 10 cal% COD, $P < 0.05$; ***, 20 cal% FOD vs 20 cal% COD, $P < 0.001$

In our study, C57B16 mice (6 to 8 weeks of age) received a standard chow for rodents with 5.3% total crude fat supplemented with refined 60% fish oil or coconut oil. Oils were given orally as 5%, 10%, or 20% of total calories per kilogram and day.

Figure 3 demonstrates blood glucose levels as percentage of diabetic controls. Lowest blood glucose was measured in the fish-fed group 60 days after the induction of diabetes. This beneficial effect was not found when streptozocin was given as a single high dose. Pancreatic insulin was nearly normal in the fish oil treated groups. Groups did not differ in pancreatic glucagon content.

We observed decreased class two antigen expression in fish oil fed multiple low-dose streptozocin-treated mice. Fish oil reduced the number of Ia-positive cells in islet sections. Subsequently, insulitis was delayed and less pronounced in the fish-fed groups.

Our current working hypothesis based on these findings is that macrophages in the islets are capable of processing proteins derived from insulin producing beta cells damaged by streptozocin. These proteins are presented as antigens to effector lymphocytes invading the islets. Thus, macrophages play a crucial role in initiating an immune-mediated destruction process of the endocrine pancreas in this model.

Omega-3 polyunsaturated fatty acids have been shown to suppress macrophage functions by inhibiting the production of biologically potent eicosanoids. We suppose that fish oil treatment interrupts the development of autoimmune diabetes on the macrophage level, i.e., at an early stage of the disease. Therefore, we believe that clinical trials with fish oil in recently diagnosed type one diabetes patients should be performed.

References

1. Prickett JD, Robinson DR, Steinberg AD (1983) Effects of dietary enrichment with eicosapentaenoic acid upon autoimmune nephritis in female NZB × NZW/F$_1$ mice. Arthritis and Rheum 26: 133–139
2. Kremer JM et al. (1987) Fish oil fatty acid supplementation in active rheumatoid arthritis. Ann Intern Med 106: 497–503

Omega-3- and Omega-6 Polyunsaturated Fatty Acids: Nutritional Needs and Dietary Recommendations

G. Wolfram

Essential fatty aids (EFA) are required for the structure of cell membranes, reproduction, growth, and the regulation of cell function via a group of hormone-like derivatives, the eicosanoids. These properties of EFA are more important than other nonessential functions [19]. EFA can be allocated to two fatty acid families according to the position of the first double bound from the methyl end at carbon 3 or carbon 6, the most important representatives being linoleic acid (C18:2 ω-6) and α-linolenic acid (C18:3 ω-3). In contrast, oleic acid (C18:1 ω-9) and its derivatives with the first double bound at carbon 9 can be synthesized in the body and are not essential.

In both EFA families 20 and 22 carbon chain length derivatives with 3, 4, 5, and 6 double bounds are produced. Linoleic acid (ω-6), α-linolenic acid (ω-3), and oleic acid (ω-9) compete for elongation and desaturation by the same enzyme system, which has preferential affinities as follows: α-linolenic > linoleic > oleic acid [9]. Arachidonic acid (AA) (C20:4 ω-6) is a principle component in the phospholipids of cell membranes and serves as a major precursor for prostaglandin and leukotriene synthesis. Eicosapentaenoic acid (EPA) (C20:5 ω-3) is the corresponding 20 carbon chain length derivative of α-linolenic acid, but it can be further converted to the docosahexaenoic acid (DHA) (C22:6 ω-3). The latter is particularly concentrated in highly active sites, e. g., the synaptic junction and the outer segments of the rods in the retina [21].

Of these five polyunsaturated fatty acids, linoleic acid is without any doubt essential [6]. Linoleic acid cannot be synthesized in man and has a defined metabolic significance. Arachidonic acid ceased to be regarded as an essential fatty acid after it was demonstrated that it could be synthesized in vivo from linoleic acid. Symptoms of linoleic acid deficiency can be divided into four groups according to Holman: diminished growth, external symptoms (i. e., in the rat tail necrosis, scaly dermatitis, and decreased pigmentation), anatomic changes in the skin, kidney, liver, lung, testis, ovary and pituitary, and physiologic changes, (increased basal metabolic rate, impaired water balance, increased fragility of cell membranes, and changes in intracellular membranes). In principle nearly all of these symptoms in animals or at least their correlates can be observed in humans. Since the first cases in babies 1958 [12] and the first case in adults 1971 [7] more than 20 patients with clinical manifestation of EFA deficiency have been observed and documented [32].

The position of α-linolenic acid as an essential nutrient was controversial [2]. Like linoleic acid, it cannot be synthesized in man, but the metabolic significance of α-linolenic acid is not quite clear. Administration of α-linolenic acid will reverse some but not all of the symptoms of EFA deficiency in the rat. For instance, reproductive failure is not reversed by α-linolenate, nor is growth retardation completely. The same holds with abnormal skin permeability. Some results can be interpreted in the sense

H. U. Klör (Ed.)
Lipoprotein Subfractions
Omega-3 Fatty Acids
© Springer-Verlag Berlin Heidelberg 1989

that α-linolenic acid may be essential in determining the polyunsaturated fatty acid composition and function of some specialized tissues, like the retina and brain [18, 25, 26, 33].

The α-linolenic acid derivatives EPA and DHA are found as structural components of brain and retinal tissue phospholipids and as precursors of the triene prostaglandins. DHA is a component of human cerebral cortex, retina, and muscle [23]. EPA is the immediate precursor of prostaglandin E3, thromboxan A3, and prostacyclin I3. Only a small amount of exogenously administered α-linolenic acid is metabolized to these two acids. In particular EPA is ingested for the most part preformed in dietary fish oils [13, 24]. The slow conversion of α-linolenic acid to the longer derivatives exhibits a special importance of EPA and DHA supplementation.

In context with ω-6 fatty acids the ω-3 fatty acids exert the following special functions. Platelet-membrane EPA is released in response to agonists; it inhibits the metabolism of AA and is converted to metabolic products (triene eicosanoids) that themselves inhibit platelet function [5, 11]. Leukotriene B4 influences the adherence of neutrophils to the arterial endothelium [16]. If the same holds for monocytes, which are to be transformed into macrophages, known as scavenger cells for plasma lipoproteins and releasing growth factors for the proliferation of arterial smooth muscle cells, a special inhibitory effect of ω-3 fatty acids on atherogenesis can be postulated. It was predicted that diets enriched in EPA will modify the contributions of leukotriene B4 to inflammatory and immunological reactions [10].

The essentialness of α-linolenic acid and of its longer derivatives EPA or DHA is supported by experiments in animals and observations in young patients. In infant rhesus monkeys after a diet deficient in ω-3 fatty acids a visual loss could be observed [21]. In 1982 Holman et al. [15] described the case of a 6-year-old girl with α-linolenic acid deficiency. She experienced distal numbness and paresthesias, weakness, periodic inability to walk, and blurring of vision. The authors suggest that α-linolenic acid respectively ω-3-polyenoic fatty acids are required for normal nerve function, at least in growing individuals. Meanwhile ω-3 fatty acid deficiency could be observed in five adults, documented by biochemical changes of fatty acid composition, but not by clinical symptoms [3, 22]. In a 90-year-old female with α-linolenic acid deficiency, the effects of ethyl α-linolenate on biosynthesis of prostanoids could be demonstrated [4].

In considering nutritional needs and dietary recommendations, one has to bear in mind that there is substantial species variability both in the metabolism of the different ω-6 and ω-3 fatty acids and in their requirements. The activities of the Δ6 and Δ5 desaturases for the interconversion of these polyunsaturated fatty acids differ in man and rat, for instance. The formation of eicosanoids from EPA is not observed in rat or swine, but is possible in rabbit and man [2o]. As man is different yet again we have to keep an open mind both with regard to ω-6 and ω-3 fatty acids and the possibility that their derivatives such as AA and EPA may deserve independent attention.

Of the α-linolenic acid ingested some is incorporated into phospholipids and cholesterol esters, while very little is elongated and eventually converted into prostaglandins: most α-linolenic acid probably is used as fuel. Of the EPA and DHA ingested most likely a greater percentage ends in eicosanoid synthesis. Therefore, different polyunsaturated fatty acids of the ω-3 series cannot be considered as similar with respect to their metabolic fate and their effects. In particular results from experiments with "Eskimo diets" may not be applicable to considerations of an α-linolenic acid containing diet, i. e., in central Europe.

Some experiments suggest that high doses of α-linolenic acid exert untoward effects, possibly inhibiting prostaglandin synthesis of the 1- and 2-series. The ratio between linoleic and α-linolenic acid in relevant experiments is such that only excessive use of linseed oil could produce them under conventional dietary conditions [22]. Still it may be considered prudent to keep the α-linolenic acid content of diet well below that of linoleic acid. On the other hand, possible adverse effects of high doses of linoleic acid on the tissue levels of long chain polyunsaturated fatty acids, especially DHA, in developing liver and brain of newborn infants are under discussion [17].

The requirement of man for ω-6 fatty acids can be fullfilled with the supply of linoleic acid. Taking into account normal linoleic acid levels and normal 20:3/20:4 ratios in lipids of serum and blood cells, the requirement for normal adults is 6–10 g linoleic acid per day or 3 energy% [27]. In infancy a similar supply of 1–3 energy% is recommended [8]. To determine the linoleic acid requirement for healthy people the amount of saturated and trans fatty acids in the diet, – which will increase the requirement – must be taken into account [30]. In patients with heavy injuries, the requirement for linoleic acid can be increased by up to the five fold the amount for healthy people [28, 29] (Fig. 1).

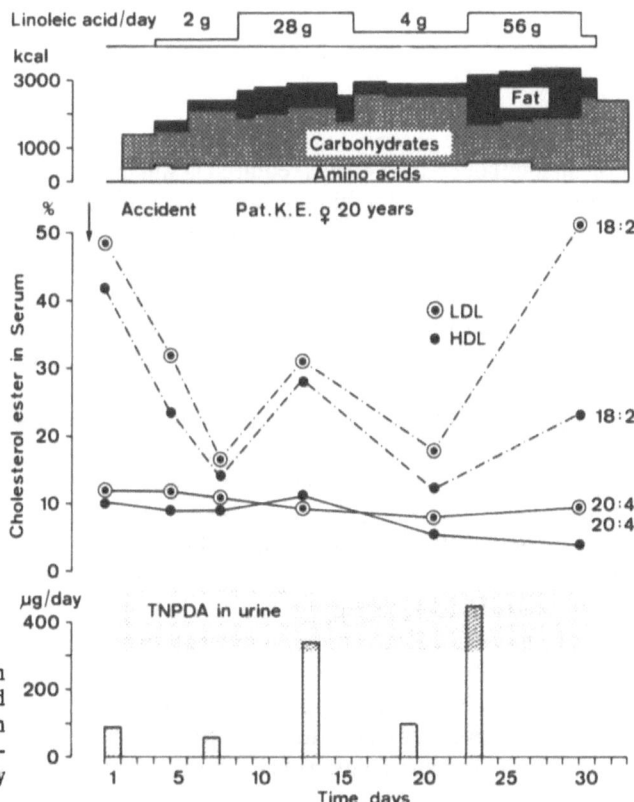

Fig. 1. ω-6 fatty acids in serum cholesterol esters and excretion of prostaglandin metabolites in urine depending on linoleic acid supply after heavy injury

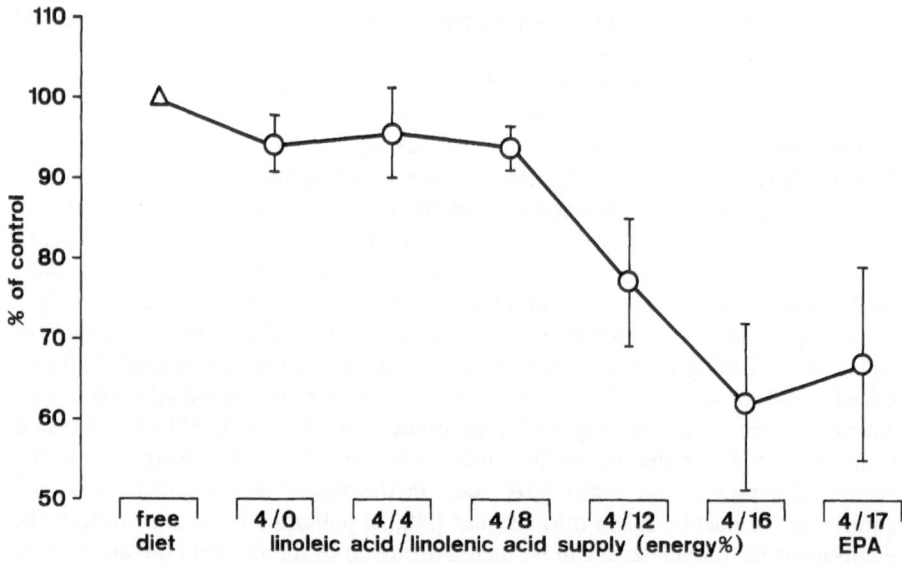

Fig. 2. ADP-induced aggregation of thrombozytes ($n = 6\,\bar{x} \pm$ S.D.)

The amount of ω-3 fatty acids required is still under discussion. At first, due to the activity of desaturases, the biological effects of α-linolenic acid and EPA in the diet were thought to be very different. In view of the platelet aggregation, a tenfold amount of α-linolenic acid is necessary to yield the effect of EPA [1] (Fig. 2). From this experience – in contrast to ω-6 fatty acids – we might need two different requirement figures for ω-3 fatty acids, a greater one for α-linolenic acid and a lower for EPA. That demands the use of a ω-3 fatty acid equivalent doses when formulating recommendations.

Holman et al. [14] estimated the requirement for α-linolenic acid in infancy to be about 0.54 energy%, in their case corresponding to 44 mg α-linolenic acid per kg body weight per day or 1.22 g α-linolenic acid per day. Calculating the requirement of adults with the 44 mg figure results in a requirement above 3 g α-linolenic acid per day. This amount seems to be very high when taking into account that the conclusions of Holman et al. [14] are based on measurements in the serum of a growing child, which possibly was to be replenished, and that the longer chain ω-3 fatty acids probably have a special importance as structural components in nerval tissue for growing individuals, but represent a by far lower need in the grown-up. In human milk, but also in tissues of man, ω-6 and ω-3 fatty acids appear in the ratio of about 5:1. In the brain this ratio is 1:1. From this point of view, and in context with a linoleic acid recommendation of 10 g per day, a recommendation of about 2 g per day α-linolenic acid for the adult may be estimated.

References

1. Adam O, Wolfram G, Zöllner N (1986) Vergleich der Wirkung von Linolsäure und Eicosapentaensäure auf die Prostaglandinbiosynthese und Thrombozytenfunktion beim Menschen. Klin Wochenschr 64: 274–280
2. Bivins BA, Bell RM, Rapp RP, Griffen WO (1983) Linoleic acid versus linolenic acid: What is essential? J Par Enteral Nutr 5: 473–478
3. Bjerve KS, Mostadt IL, Thoresen L (1987) Alpha-linolenic acid deficiency in patients on long-term gastric-tube feeding: estimation of linolenic acid and long-chain unsaturated n-3 fatty acid requirement in man. Am J Clin Nutr 77: 45–66
4. Bjerve KS, Fischer S, Alme K (1987) Alpha-linolenic acid deficiency in man: effect of ethyl linolenate on plasma and erythrocyte fatty acid composition and biosynthesis of prostanoids. Am J Clin Nutr 46: 570–576
5. Budowski P, Crawford MA (1985) Linolenic acid as a regulator of the metabolism of arachidonic acid: dietary implications of the ratio, n-6:n-3 fatty acids. Proc Nutr Soc 44: 221–229
6. Burr GO, Burr MM (1929) A new deficiency disease produced by the rigid exclusion of fat from the diet. J Biol Chem 82: 345–367
7. Collins FD, Sinclair AJ, Royle JP, Coats DA, Maynard AT, Leonard RF (1971) Plasma lipids in human linoleic acid deficiency. Nutr Metabol 13: 150–167
8. Crawford MA, Hassam AG, Rivers JPW (1978) Essential fatty acid requirement in infancy. A J Clin Nutr 31: 2181–2185
9. Galli C, Agradi E, Paoletti R (1974) The (n-6) pentaene: (n-3) hexaene fatty acid ratio as an index of linolenic acid deficiency. Biochimica et Biophysica Acta 369: 142–145
10. Goldman DW, Picket WC, Goetzl EJ (1983) Human neutrophil chemotactic and degranulating activities of leukotriene B5 (LTB5) derived from eicosapentaenoic acid. Biochem Biophys Res Comm 117: 282–288
11. Goodnight SH, Harris WS, Connor WE, Illingworth DR (1982) Polyunsaturated fatty acids, hyperlipidemia, and thrombosis. Arteriosclerosis 2: 87–113
12. Hansen AE, Haggard ME, Boelsche AN, Adam DJD, Wiese HF (1958) Essential fatty acids in infant nutrition. III. Clinical manifestations of linoleic acid deficiency. J Nutrition 4: 565–576
13. Hepburn F, Exler J, Weihrauch J (1986) Provisional tables on the content of omega-3 fatty acids and other fat components of selected foods. J Amer Dietet Ass 86: 788–793
14. Holman RT, Caster WO, Wiese HF (1964) The essential fatty acid requirement of infants and the assessment of their dietary intake of linoleate by serum fatty acid analysis. Am J Clin Nutr 14: 70–75
15. Holman RT, Johnson SB, Hatch TF (1982) A case of human linolenic acid deficiency involving neurological abnormalities. Am J Clin Nutr 35: 617–623
16. Hoover RL, Karnovsky MJ, Austen KF, Corey EJ, Lewis RA (1984) Leukotriene B4 action on endothelium mediates angmented neutrophil/endothelial adhesion. Proc Natl Acad Sci USA 81: 2191–2193
17. Martinez M, Ballabriga A (1987) Effects of parenteral nutrition with high doses of linoleate on the developing human liver and brain. Lipids 22: 133–138
18. Lamptey MS and Walker BL (1976) A possible essential role for dietary linolenic acid in the development of the young rat. J Nutrition 106: 86–93
19. Mead JF (1984) The non-eicosanoid functions of the essential fatty acids. J Lipid Res 25: 1517–1521
20. Movita I, Takahashi R, Saito Y, Murota S (1983) Thrombosis Res 31: 211–217
21. Neuringer M, Connor WE, Van Petten C, Barstad L (1984) Dietary omega-3 fatty acid deficiency and visual loss in infant Rhesus monkeys. J Clin Invest 73: 272–276
22. Stein TP, Marino PL, Harner RN (1986) Combined EFA deficiency in a patient on long-term TPN. Nutrition Reviews 44: 301–305
23. Svennerholm L (1968) Distribution and fatty acid composition of phosphoglycerides in normal human brain. J Lipid Res 9: 570–579
24. Taylor G, Gibney MJ and Morgan JB (1979) Haemostatic function and polyunsaturated fatty acids. Lancet II, 1378

25. Tinoco J, Babcock R, Hincenbergs I, Medwadowski B, Miljanich P and Williams MA (1979) Linolenic acid deficiency. Lipids 14: 166–173
26. Wheeler TG, Benolken RM, Anderson RE (1975) Visual membranes: specificity of fatty acid precursors for the electrical response to illumination. Science 188: 1312–1314
27. Wolfram G, Zöllner N (1971) Der Linolsäurebedarf des Menschen. Wiss Veröff Dt Ges für Ernährung 22: 51–60, Steinkopff Verlag Darmstadt
28. Wolfram G, Eckart J, Walther B, Zöllner N (1978) Factors influencing essential fatty acid requirement in total parenteral nutrition. J Parent Ent Nutr 2: 634–639
29. Wolfram G, Eckart J (1983) Die essentiellen Fettsäuren im Plasma von Schwerverletzten. Klin Wochenschr 61: 1181–1189
30. Wolfram G, Adam O, Zöllner N (1984) Wirkung der Linol- und Linolensäure auf die Prostaglandinbildung und die Nierenfunktion beim Menschen. fette-seifen-anstrichmittel 5: 180–183
31. Wolfram G, Adam O, Zöllner N (1986) Pain, prostaglandins, and food lipids. Bibl Nutr Dieta 38: 112–119
32. Wolfram G (1987) Essentielle Fettsäuren in der parenteralen Ernährung. Infusionstherapie 14: 20–28
33. Yamamoto N, Saitoh M, Moriuchi A, Nomura M (1987) Effect of dietary α-linolenate/linoleate balance on brain lipid compositions and learning ability of rats. J Lipid Res 28: 144–151

Omega-3 Fatty Acid Treatment of Hyperlipidemia: Efficacy and Mechanism of Action

H. U. KLÖR, and C. H. LULEY

Recent studies by Bang and Dyerberg [1] have stimulated interest in the metabolism of omega-3 fatty acids and have suggested a link between the ingestion of these fatty acids in a diet and the low death rate from atherosclerotic disease in Eskimos. In Japan, where fish consumption has traditionally been high, a concomitant shift in tissue lipid consumption favouring omega-3 polyunsaturated fatty acids (PUFA) has been interpreted as a reason for the relatively low incidence of cardiovascular disease [1]. On analyzing the Eskimo diet, it became clear that the consumption of omega-3 PUFA is much higher, besides a 50% reduction of saturated fat and a relatively high content of monounsaturated fat with a chain length of more than 18 carbon atoms. The total fat intake of the Eskimos is in the order of 40% of total calories per day, as high a proportion as in Western diets. In addition, daily cholesterol intake averages almost 800 mg, even higher than in most Western diets.

Comparing lipid and lipoprotein levels of Greenland Eskimos and Danes, Dyerberg and Bang [2] found significantly lower LDL and VLDL concentrations in Eskimos, leading to drastically lower triglyceride and total plasma cholesterol concentrations. The HDL levels were about the same.

Between 1956 and 1963 7 studies of fish oil feeding were carried out in normal volunteers [3–9]. Although they varied in the kinds of subjects studied, in the degree of dietary control and in the source of fish oil, there was good agreement that fish oils were at least as hypocholesterolemic as polyunsaturated vegetable oils. Two interesting features of these studies were not appreciated at the time: Since natural, unrefined fish oils contain large amounts of cholesterol (300–500 mg/dl) and vegetable oils contain none, the majority of investigators fed higher levels of cholesterol during the fish oil phase than during the vegetable oil phase. Also, daily intake of omega-6 fatty acids, even with the fish oil-enriched diets, was greater than the intake of omega-3 fatty acids, and yet similar or greater reductions in plasma cholesterol levels occurred from omega-3 fatty acids. These reductions occurred when omega-3 fatty acids constituted from 1% to 8% of total calories. In light of the fact that linoleic acid intakes of 15%–20% of calories were needed to achieve similar depressions in plasma cholesterol levels, the dietary omega-3 fatty acids were roughly 2–5 times more potent than the omega-6 PUFA.

Dramatic reductions in the concentrations of plasma triglycerides and VLDL have been observed in both normolipidemic [10–12] and hyperlipidemic subjects [3–13] fed diets supplemented with fish oils. Harris et al. [12] compared the effect of salmon oil and vegetable oil and found that plasma cholesterol levels were reduced similarly with both salmon oil-rich and vegetable oil-rich diets. In contrast, plasma triglyceride levels fell 33% in the salmon oil diet, but were unchanged after the vegetable oil diet.

H. U. Klör (Ed.)
Lipoprotein Subfractions
Omega-3 Fatty Acids
© Springer-Verlag Berlin Heidelberg 1989

VLDL concentrations fell 50% and LDL concentrations 60% without any change in HDL concentration. In a number of recent studies in hyperlipoproteinemic patients, the significant fall of VLDL and, in some groups, also of LDL was confirmed. The most dramatic effects occurred in type V hyperlipoproteinemia, which is characterized by elevated VLDL and by fasting chylomicronemia. Phillipson and colleagues [13] reported triglyceride reductions of 79% and cholesterol decreases of 45% in this group of patients. Giving a vegetable oil to these patients produced a rapid and significant rise in plasma triglyceride levels. Similar results in type V hyperlipoproteinemia have been reported by Sanders et al. [14] and Simons et al. [15].

In contrast to extensive studies on the mechanism of action of saturated fatty acids and omega-6 PUFA there are only a few studies on the mechanism of action of omega-3 PUFA. Illingworth et al. [16] showed in a group of seven healthy volunteers that omega-3 PUFA administration caused a reduction of total cholesterol from 160 to 124 mg/dl and of LDL from 103 to 82 mg/dl. Triglyceride levels fell by almost 50% from 91 to 52 mg/dl. In these normal subjects, kinetic studies of iodinated LDL metabolism disclosed a significantly lower rate of synthesis of LDL apolipoprotein B (ApoB) on the omega-3 diet. In contrast, the fractional catabolic rate of LDL was similar in both diets. These authors concluded that dietary omega-3 PUFA lowered plasma LDL in normal human subjects by reducing the rate of synthesis of ApoB.

Nestel and coworkers [17] recently showed that the reason for the reduced VLDL concentrations was that VLDL synthesis was markedly reduced after 3 weeks of fish oil as compared to a safflower oil diet. There was also a significant reduction of daily production of VLDL triglyceride, as calculated from radiolabeled glycerol injection studies. The fractional removal rate as a measure for VLDL catabolism was not consistently affected, indicating that the plasma lipolytic system was probably not activated. In a recent experiment, Harris and coworkers [18] were able to show that the hypertriglyceridemia induced by high carbohydrate intake could be prevented by dietary omega-3 PUFA. When a high-carbohydrate diet was given to normal volunteers, the plasma triglyceride level rose from 105 to 194 mg/dl. When fish oil was given, the plasma triglyceride levels fell from 194 to 75 mg/dl, and the VLDL triglyceride and cholesterol levels were reduced from 156 to 34 and from 34 to 12 mg/dl respectively. These effects were noted after only 2 or 3 days of fish oil diet, indicating an extremely rapid onset of the fish oil effect.

As mentioned above, evaluation of the Eskimo diet showed a fairly high dietary intake of cholesterol in the presence of very low average plasma cholesterol and LDL cholesterol level [19]. This raises the question of whether omega-3 PUFA might be able to counteract the hypercholesterolemic effect of cholesterol. In a recent study by Nestel [20] this question was addressed in six normolipidemic subjects, who received first a Western diet, then a fish oil-enriched diet providing approximately 13 g omega-3 PUFA per day besides a lowered cholesterol and lowered saturated fat content. Switching to that diet resulted in a 20% decrease of plasma cholesterol, VLDL and LDL cholesterol as well as a highly significant decrease in HDL cholesterol. Plasma triglycerides decreased by more than 60%. Maintaining that same diet, but adding 800 mg cholesterol per day in the form of egg yolk, did not lead to a substantial rise in the plasma lipid or lipoprotein parameters measured. Although the dietary periods were perhaps not long enough (3 weeks) and too many variables were changed at the same time (saturated fat, cholesterol content, fish oil), this study still raises the interesting

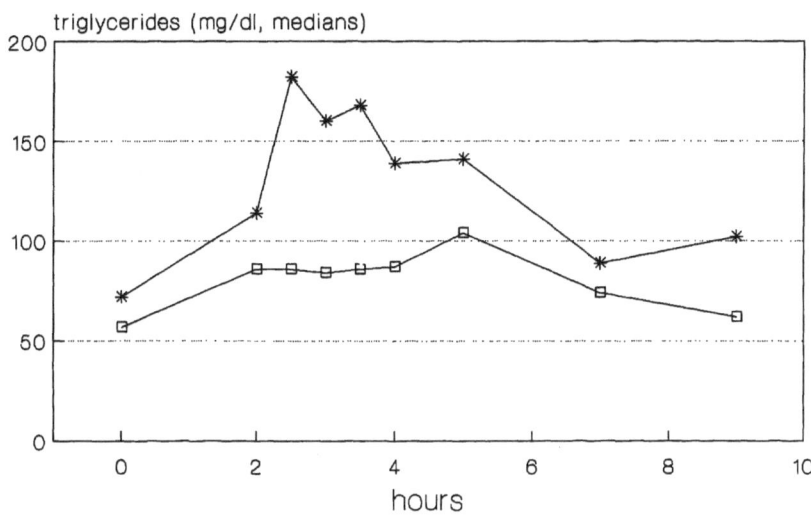

Fig. 1. The results of fat load (with 100 g butter) before (*) and after (□) a 4-week period of omega-3 PUFA supplementation

question of whether pure supplementation with omega-3 PUFA in relatively small amounts might be able to counteract the hypercholesterolemic effect of food items containing saturated fat and cholesterol.

We recently studied the effect of supplementation of an ordinary Wester diet with 8 g omega-3 PUFA in the form of purified fish oil capsules in 20 healthy volunteers. In particular, the rise in plasma triglycerides induced by an oral fat load was studied before and after a 4-week period of omega-3 PUFA supplementation. As expected, a fat load consisting of 100 g butter led to a significant postprandial increase of trigly-ceride over a period of 5–7 h. However, only half of the participants showed a very significant rise in triglyceride of close to 100% postprandially. After 4 weeks of fish oil capsule treatment, the fat load with butter was repeated. This time, none of the participants showed any significant increase in postprandial triglycerides (Fig. 1).

When a fat load consisting of 100 g fish oil (60 g omega-3 PUFA) was given, there was no increase in postprandial triglyceride values, indicating an apparent lack of response to the large load of omega-3 PUFA. In contrast to the large fat load with butter, significant diarrhea developed in all 20 participants, with up to 10 bowel movements over the next 24 h. The first bowel movement occurred already 5–7 h after fat ingestion, indicating a much shortened intestinal transit time due to maldiges-tion and/or malabsorption. Neither the butter load nor an equivalent fat load with 100 g safflower oil rich in omega-5 PUFA produced such an effect.

When fecal fat excretion (Fig. 2) was determined over the 24-h period following the ingestion of butter, safflower oil or fish oil before and after the 4-week period of fish oil capsule treatment, there were clear indications that the ingestion of large quan-tities of fish oil in form of a fat load caused severe steatorrhea. This was particularly evident after the treatment period with fish oil capsules.

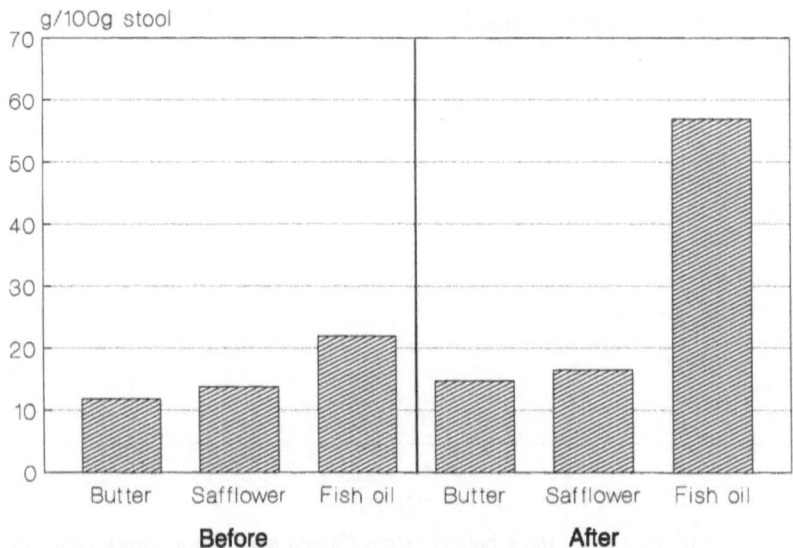

Fig. 2. Fecal fat excretion over a 24-h period following the ingestion of butter, safflower oil or fish oil before and after a 4-week period of fish,oil capsule treatment

We had hypothesized that a possible mechanism leading to an attenuated response to an acute fat load of saturated fat might be a temporary retention of triglycerides in the intestinal mucosa during the process of chylomicron formation and release. In order to evaluate that possibility we took small intestinal biopsies via an upper endoscopy 5 h after the beginning of the fat load.

Fig. 3 shows the mucosal concentrations of triglyceride, cholesterol ester and free cholesterol as analyzed by gas chromatography. The mucosal concentration of these lipids was compared in the fasting state, after the butter load and before the fish oil capsule treatment, after the butter load following a 4-week period of omega-3 PUFA treatment, and after the large fish oil load. The large fish oil load caused a significant increase – as might be expected – of mucosal triglyceride. However, the mucosal cholesterol ester content did not increase at all as compared to the fasting state. The free cholesterol remained the same as well. When comparing the mucosal lipid content after the butter load before and following the omega-3 PUFA capsule treatment there was no change in free cholesterol concentration. It was interesting to note that the mucosal triglyceride content was somewhat higher when the butter load was given after the fish oil capsule treatment. Such a tendency could also be observed in the mucosal cholesterol esters. Although these data are not conclusive they seem to indicate that some retention of intestinal triglyceride and cholesterol ester might occur after pretreatment with low-dose omega-3 PUFA.

When comparing the plasma triglyceride results shown in Fig. 1 and the mucosal triglyceride concentrations shown in Fig. 3 at 5 h after the fat load, it is interesting to note that the plasma triglyceride is highest at that time. This could be interpreted as a

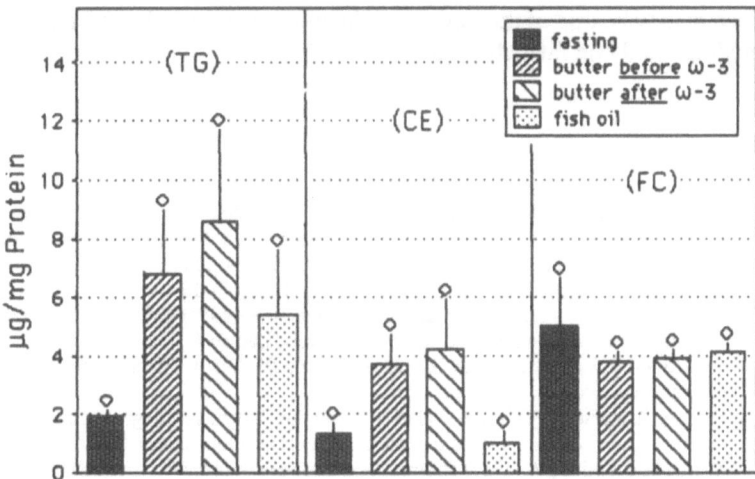

Fig. 3. The mucosal concentrations of triglyceride *(TG)*, cholesterol esters *(CE)* and free cholesterol *(FC)* in the fasting state, following butter loads before and after omega-3 PUFA treatment, and following a fish oil load

reflection of a delayed release of stored mucosal triglyceride in the form of chylomicrons. Indeed, chylomicron triglyceride concentration at that time point was higher than at earlier time points after fish oil capsule treatment. Without fish oil capsules given before the acute butter load the chylomicron triglyceride concentration reached its peak at 3 h after the fat load and was significantly lower at 5 h.

In conclusion, our preliminary results indicate that ingestion of large quantities of omega-3 PUFA (60 g at a time) do not induce postprandial hypertriglyceridemia at all. One of the apparent reasons for this total lack of response seems to be the induction of either maldigestion or malabsorption and subsequent steatorrhea. The mechanism of this malassimilation is unclear. The analysis of mucosal lipid content at a relatively late time point in the process of lipid absorption and processing in the mucosa seems to indicate that triglyceride synthesized from the fish oil accumulates to some extent in the mucosa and is not released in the form of chylomicron triglyceride. The total lack of mucosal cholesterol ester may be interpreted as the consequence of malabsorption of luminal cholesterol during the large fish oil load.

The chronic administration of small quantities of omega-3 PUFA attenuates the postprandial response to saturated fat. Our mucosal lipid studies seem to indicate that some retention of saturated triglyceride might occur in the intestinal mucosa before the triglyceride is released in the form of chylomicrons. This delayed release might improve the substrate situation for the intravascular lipolytic system and thereby help to maintain a relatively low postprandial triglyceride level. This effect of chronic omega-3 PUFA administration may be responsible for the triglyceride-lowering effect seen in type V hyperlipoproteinemia, where chylomicron concentrations are very high even in fasting plasma. The observation that chronic ingestion of omega-3 PUFA can attenuate the postprandial lipemia induced by saturated fat merits confirmation in a larger group of individuals over a prolonged period of time, because postprandial lipemia may be one of the key events in atherogenesis in Western populations living predominantly on fat-rich diets.

References

1. Bang HO, Dyerberg J (1980) Lipid metabolism and ischemic heart disease in Greenland eskimos. In: Draper HH (ed) Advanced nutrition research, vol 3. Plenum Press New York, pp 1–22
2. Dyerberg J, Bang HO (1982) A hypothesis on the development of acute myocardial infarction in Greenlanders. Scand J Clin Lab Invest 42 [Suppl 161]: 7–13
3. Kingsbury KJ, Morgan DM, Aylott C, Emmerson R (1961) Effects of ethyl arachidonate, cod liver oil and corn oil on plasma cholesterol levels. Lancet 1: 739
4. Bronte-Stewart B, Antonis A, Easles L, Brock JF (1956) Effects of feeding different fats on serum cholesterol levels. Lancet 1: 521
5. Keys A, Anderson JT, Grande F (1957) "Essential" fatty acids: degree of unsaturation and effects of corn (maize) oil on the serum cholesterol level in man. Lancet 1: 66
6. Worne HE, Smith SW (1959) Effects of certain pure long chain polyunsaturated fatty acid esters on blood lipids of man. Am J Med Sci 237: 710
7. Kinsell LW, Michaels GD, Walker G, Visintine RE (1961) The effect of a fish-oil fraction on plasma lipids. Diabetes 10: 316
8. Kingsbury KJ, Morgan DM, Aylott C, Emmerson R (1961) Effects of ethyl arachidonate, cod liver and corn oil on plasma cholesterol levels. Lancet I: 739
9. Imaichi K, Michaels GD, Gunning G et al. (1963) Studies with the use of fish oil fractions in human subjects. Am J Clin Nutr 13: 158
10. Bronsegeest-Schoute HC, van Gent CM, Luten JB et al. (1981) The effects of various intakes of omega-3 fatty acids on the blood lipid composition in healthy human subjects. Am J Clin Nutr 34: 1752
11. Sanders TB, Vickers M, Haines AP (1981) Effect on blood lipids and haemostasis of a supplement of cod liver oil, rich in eicosapentaenoic and docosahexaenoic acids, in healthy young men. Clin Sci 61: 317
12. Harris WS, Connor WE (1980) The effects of salmon oil upon plasma lipids, lipoproteins and triglyceride clearance. Trans Assoc Am Physicians 43: 14
13. Phillipson BE, Rothrock DW, Connor WE et al. (1985) Reduction of plasma lipids, lipoproteins and apoproteins by dietary fish oils in patients with hypertriglyceridemia. N Engl J Med 312: 1210–1216
14. Sanders T, Sullivan DR, Reeve J, Thompson G (1985) Triglyceride lowering effect of marine polyunsaturates in patients with hypertriglyceridemia. Arteriosclerosis 5: 459–465
15. Simons LA, Hickie JB, Balasubramaniam S (1985) On the effect of dietary n-3 fatty acids (Maxepa) on plasma lipids and lipoproteins in patients with hyperlipidemia. Atherosclerosis 54: 75–87
16. Illingworth R, Harris WS, Connor WE (1984) Inhibition of low density lipoprotein synthesis by dietary omega-3 fatty acids in humans. Arteriosclerosis 4: 270
17. Nestel P, Connor WE, Reardon MF et al. (1984) Suppression by diets rich in fish oil of very low density lipoprotein production in man. J Clin Invest 74: 82–89
18. Harris WS, Connor WE, Inteles SB, Illingworth R (1984) Dietary omega-3 fatty acids prevent carbohydrate-induced hypertriglyceridemia. Metabolism 33: 1016–1019
19. Dyerberg J (1986) Linolenate-derived polyunsaturated fatty acids and prevention of atherosclerosis. Nutr Rev 44: 125–134
20. Nestel PJ (1986) Fish oil attenuates the cholesterol induced rise in lipoprotein cholesterol. Am J Clin Nutr 43: 752–757

Subject Index